The ABC's of
Advanced Prostate Cancer

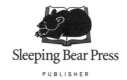

Sleeping Bear Press

PUBLISHER

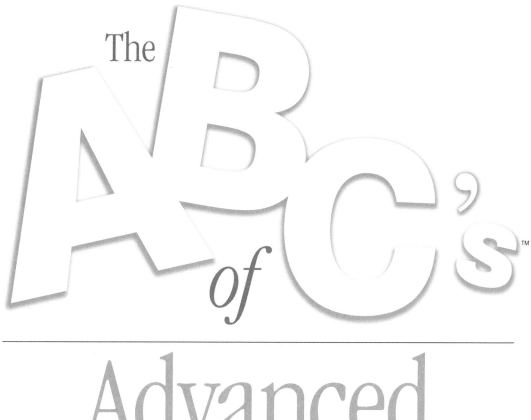

The ABC's of

Advanced

Prostate Cancer

By Mark A. Moyad, M.P.H. and Kenneth J. Pienta, M.D.

Copyright 2000 Mark Moyad, M.P.H. and Kenneth J. Pienta, M.D.
Illustrations by Patrick J. Gloria

Sleeping Bear Press
310 North Main, Suite 300
P.O. Box 20
Chelsea, Michigan 48118
www.sleepingbearpress.com

Printed and bound in The United States.
10 9 8 7 6 5 4 3 2 1

Moyad, Mark A.,
ABC's of advanced prostate cancer / by Mark A. Moyad and
Kenneth J. Pienta.
p. cm.
"A companion book to The ABC's of nutrition & supplements"–Cover.
ISBN 1-886947-68-6
1. Prostate–Cancer–Popular works.
I. Pienta, Kenneth J.
II. Title: ABC's of nutrition and supplements for prostate cancer.
RC280. P7M687 2000
616.99' 463–DC21

99-14167
CIP

In 1992, I graduated from the University of South Florida College of Public Health with a Master's degree. Public Health is synonymous with prevention, a fact I would never ever forget. I was able to travel the world and see individuals with terrible diseases that were easily preventable with the right amount of money and knowledge. When I returned home from my travels I was convinced that these third world problems did not apply to more advanced countries like the United States, but I was simply wrong. Cancer, heart disease—these chronic diseases can be prevented to a large degree but it is not easy. We have to invest in our researchers—give them the tools that will allow them to find out exactly what you and I can do to prevent these terrible diseases from taking the lives of so many individuals. Our researchers are like soldiers who have been recruited (voluntarily) to fight an international war; however, they have only been given a pocketknife to battle a gigantic enemy. Is this really all we can do right now? I am 100% convinced that if given the resources and money to buy more than a pocketknife we can wipe out these enemies such as cancer and do so in a short amount of time. At this very moment, we have the dedicated individuals, minds, and technology; every piece of the puzzle is in place to solve this mystery. Only one essential piece is missing—and unfortunately it is in the form of a dollar sign. Once the funding is available, the mystery of prostate cancer will be solved.

In 1997, Ken Pienta came into my office to talk. My immediate reaction was, "Can this guy really be a doctor? He looks like he's late for his 10th grade geometry class!" I was surprised he wanted to see me, because although I had not worked with him, I of course knew of his reputation. He's known as "the advanced prostate cancer doctor at the University of Michigan." He was brief but to the point with only one question, "Have you ever considered coauthoring a book on advanced prostate cancer? It's a real problem, an epidemic in many ways, and books give patients very little information regarding this subject." I told him that I had never considered writing such a book because we covered the subject in my first book, *The ABCs of Prostate Cancer*. He persisted, "Yes, but you see there was only a chapter or two in your book on advanced prostate cancer. I'm talking about an entire book dedicated to the subject."

I couldn't decide if I was honored or upset that Dr. Pienta asked me to be a part of this project, because I really believed (at the time) there was no need for such a book. However, before I officially said "No" to his unique request I decided to do a little homework. To make a long story short, I was completely amazed at what I learned. When cancer leaves, or threatens to leave, the prostate patients enter an entirely new realm of many *more* choices and much *more* confusion.

Hormonal therapy, chemotherapy, surgery, alternative medicines, pain management, etc., and on and on it goes. Depending on whom you talk to, about 50% of the men diagnosed with prostate cancer will eventually have some stage of advanced disease. At least 40,000 men in the United States alone die from this disease every year, and all of them from an advanced stage.

I wasted little time after my educational session on advanced disease before I told Dr. Pienta that I would be honored to write such a book with him. Our work, *The ABC's of Advanced Prostate Cancer*, is the first of its kind in medicine for these patients. To Ken Pienta I owe a debt of gratitude, he ignited a spark within me for this work. It is truly a labor of love. Ken deserves all the credit for beginning this work.

It was a tough, tough year. We both wanted a book that was the best source of its kind. Late night meetings, weekends, cellular calls at all hours..."It has to be the best, second to nothing" became our mantra. The problem was that there were no examples for us to follow. When I did *The ABCs of Prostate Cancer* there were many previous books published on the subject that I was able to examine and digest before creating the final work. This disease has no easy solutions and nothing at all written on the topic. We had to actually "create the wheel" this time.

It is my hope that *The ABC's of Advanced Prostate Cancer* becomes an invaluable resource for you, your family, your friends, loved ones, and doctor. I also hope that it will have a short life. I dream one day that my future children will ask "Daddy, what is advanced prostate cancer?" And I will respond, "Kids, many years ago there was a big, big problem called prostate cancer. We found a cure though, and now no one dies of this disease anymore. So don't worry about it, just go in the kitchen and drink the rest of your soy milk, grab your supplements and lunch bags (filled with fruits and vegetables), and I'll take you to school."

I will leave you with what I tell all my patients, "Individual knowledge and empowerment is the first step toward a successful outcome." After reading this book, I guarantee that you will have taken that first step.

Sincerely,
Mark A. Moyad, M.P.H.

Many books have been written about what a patient needs to know about the diagnosis and treatment of prostate cancer. Unfortunately, these books use the majority of their pages to tell patients how to make decisions about localized prostate cancer (cancer which has not spread beyond the confines of the prostate gland). *The ABC's of Advanced Prostate Cancer* is meant to be a comprehensive guide for patients who want to understand the important aspects of advanced prostate cancer and how it impacts them. It explains the anatomy, tests involved in diagnosis, and various treatments for cancer when it is no longer confined to the gland itself.

In 1991, I joined the faculty of Wayne State University Medical School in Detroit, Michigan. In 1994, I moved to the University of Michigan in Ann Arbor, where I am a Professor of Medicine and Surgery. As the Director of the Urologic Oncology Program for the University of Michigan Comprehensive Cancer Center, I guide an active laboratory developing new therapies for advanced, hormone-refractory prostate cancer, as well as investigate why prostate cancer metastasizes (or spreads) so often to the bones. I also have an active clinical practice taking care of men with hormone refractory prostate cancer. A wonderful team helps accomplish these things. Since 1991, we and others have developed several active regimens that we believe are helping people with advanced prostate cancer live longer and with a better quality of life. Cancer wears many faces over time. It can appear to lay dormant and then, all of a sudden, start to grow quickly. It can shrink dramatically with treatment, and then remain in remission or grow back just as quickly. The treatment of advanced prostate cancer often lies in understanding when to treat, when not to treat, and/or when to change therapy. Despite the advances in the last 10 years, there are still many unanswered questions. Our most recent combination of medicines helps two-thirds of patients achieve at least a temporary remission, and we are aiming for even higher response rates in an effort to find a cure for advanced, hormone-refractory prostate cancer.

This is an exciting time for us in the field of prostate cancer research and treatment. Prostate cancer researchers around the world are actively pursuing treatment strategies that we hope will lead to a cure of metastatic prostate cancer. These include new chemotherapies, new antimetastasis strategies, new vaccine therapies, as well as new ways to attack the tumor by targeting the blood vessels, which feed the tumor. We will bring these theories to the clinic as soon as possible. In the meantime, advanced prostate cancer exists as a major health problem. If you or someone you love has it or is concerned about it, this book is designed to serve as a guide for understanding this disease and what you can do about it right now.

In closing, I would like to thank my coauthor Mark Moyad, who was the driving force behind this book. I also thank the staff at Sleeping Bear Press for helping us make *The ABC's of Advanced Prostate Cancer* into what we believe is a great book that patients and their families will find helpful.

I salute Don Coffey—mentor, friend, and a driving force in prostate cancer research in this country for 40 years. I am grateful beyond words to my family for their support. And finally, as much as anyone, I dedicate this book to Gerald Malley:

> He lived a good life.
> He fought the good fight.
> He inspired us all.
> We miss you.

> Sincerely,
> Kenneth J. Pienta, M.D.

1

The Basics: Understanding Advanced Prostate Cancer

In this chapter:

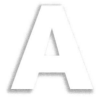

What Should I Know about Prostate Cancer and Advanced Prostate Cancer?

How Does Prostate Cancer Become Advanced?

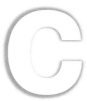

How Can I Tell If I Have Advanced Prostate Cancer? What Are the Symptoms?

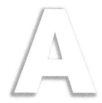

What Should I Know about Prostate Cancer and Advanced Prostate Cancer?

What is the Number 1 cancer diagnosed in men today? Colon cancer? Lung cancer? Skin cancer?

No, it's prostate cancer. In fact:

► Prostate cancer accounts for more than 40% of all the cancers diagnosed in men.

► Since 1998, nearly 200,000 men a year have been diagnosed with prostate cancer in the United States. That trend is expected to continue at least through the year 2002.

► 1 out of 8 men will be diagnosed with prostate cancer in their lifetime.

► Every three minutes, someone is diagnosed with prostate cancer.

Cancer Incidence			
Men		**Women**	
Prostate	43%	Breast	30%
Lung	12%	Lung	13%
Colon & Rectum	8.5%	Colon & Rectum	11%
Bladder	5%	Uterus	6%
Non-Hodgkin's Lymphoma	4%	Ovary	4.5%
Melanoma (skin cancer)	3%	Non-Hodgkin's Lymphoma	4%
Oral Cavity (mouth & throat)	3%	Melanoma (skin cancer)	3%
Kidney	2%	Bladder	2.5%
Leukemia	2%	Cervix	2%
Stomach	2%	Pancreas	2%

Cancer Mortality			
Men		**Women**	
Lung	32%	Lung	25%
Prostate	14%	Breast	16.5%
Colon & Rectum	9%	Colon & Rectum	10.5%
Pancreas	4.5%	Pancreas	5.5%
Non-Hodgkin's Lymphoma	4%	Ovary	5%
Leukemia	4%	Non-Hodgkin's Lymphoma	4%
Esophagus	3%	Leukemia	3.5%
Stomach	3%	Uterus	2%
Bladder	2.5%	Brain	2%
Liver	2.5%	Stomach	2%

The point, of course, is that prostate cancer is a fairly common disease. More important, however, is that 30% to 40% of men with prostate cancer have some type of "advanced" or "metastatic" cancer at the time of diagnosis. This means it is no longer only in the prostate and may eventually be found in other parts of the body.

Prostate cancer is not only increasingly common, it's also serious. Consider that:
► Prostate cancer is the Number 2 cancer killer of men in the United States, second only to lung cancer.
► In 1973, 18,830 American men died of prostate cancer. By 1998, that figure had grown to about 40,000 per year, and in the next few years, the toll is expected to reach more than 45,000 men annually.
► Someone dies of prostate cancer in the United States every 13 minutes.
► Deaths due to prostate cancer are also increasing in other parts of the world, such as Australia, Europe, Japan, and Russia.

The growing number of deaths from prostate cancer is not simply the result of a growing population. Over the last 25 years, the prostate cancer death rate—a figure that is independent of population size—has increased 25%. In other words, a greater percentage of men are dying from prostate cancer than ever before. There is some evidence that the death rate has been declining in the last few years, but until that trend continues for some time, we will be faced with more and more cases of—and deaths from—prostate cancer.

Basically, the men who die of prostate cancer die of advanced prostate cancer. We believe that the subject of advanced prostate cancer deserves an in-depth

Predictions of Prostate Cancer Deaths

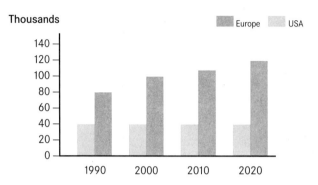

Thousands

Europe USA

The Problem of Advanced Prostate Cancer

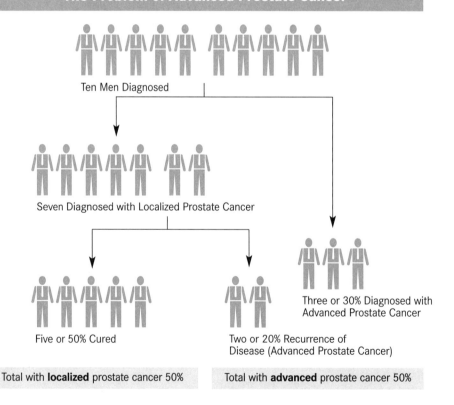

Ten Men Diagnosed

Seven Diagnosed with Localized Prostate Cancer

Five or 50% Cured

Two or 20% Recurrence of Disease (Advanced Prostate Cancer)

Three or 30% Diagnosed with Advanced Prostate Cancer

Total with **localized** prostate cancer 50%

Total with **advanced** prostate cancer 50%

look, one that separates it from the more general discussions of localized prostate cancer. That is why we have written this book.

There are some basic facts and concepts about the prostate and prostate cancer that will help you get the most out of this book. As we explore the topic of advanced prostate cancer, we will assume that you have a pretty good understanding of some of those basic facts, such as:

▶ The location and size of the prostate (it's about the size of a walnut).
▶ Some of the tests used to diagnose prostate cancer, such as the PSA test.
▶ The grading and stages of prostate cancer.
▶ Some of the treatment options for localized cancer.

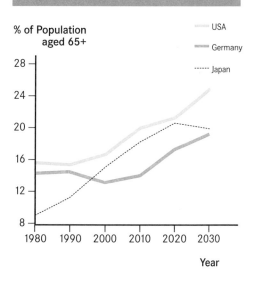

% of Population Aged 65+

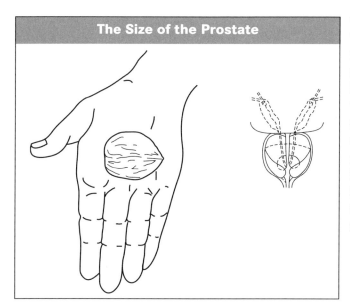

The Size of the Prostate

Overall, this book is for men who not only want to know more about prostate cancer in general, but who have had localized cancer and are worried about treatment and possible progression— or those who have advanced prostate cancer. Just as important, it is also written for the family and friends of those men who want to learn more about the disease.

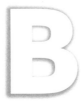

How Does Prostate Cancer Become Advanced?

There is no simple answer to that question—we are not exactly sure how or why men get prostate cancer. Advanced prostate cancer begins, of course, with localized prostate cancer that spreads after treatment has failed or because the cancer was not diagnosed in the localized stages. There are several major risk factors associated with prostate cancer in general, including age, geographic location, race, family history, and hormone levels. Many of these factors can't be controlled or avoided, but there are a few you can do something about. Let's take a look at both the nonpreventable and the preventable risk factors.

Nonpreventable Risk Factors

Age

The biggest risk factor for prostate cancer is clearly a man's age. In fact, almost 80% of the men diagnosed with prostate cancer are 65 years of age or older. Few men in their twenties are diagnosed with prostate cancer, but about 10% to 20% of men in their 30s have the disease. By age 50, nearly 1 out of 3 men will have prostate cancer. By age 70, that climbs to about 70%; by age 80, to just under 80%; and by age 90, to about—you guessed it—90%. The disease is so common in elderly men, who typically have other health problems as well, that doctors often say, "You are more likely to die *with* prostate cancer than *from* prostate cancer." That's true, but that saying should not lead anyone to become complacent about the disease. Remember: One of eight men will develop prostate cancer that affects his life and approximately one-third of those men will develop advanced prostate cancer. It's the Number 2 cancer killer of men!

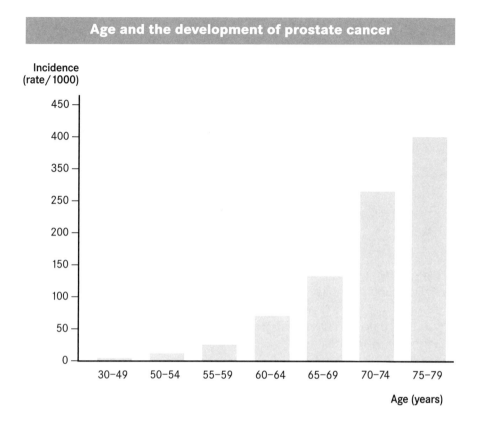

Family history

In the United States, the average man's risk of one day having prostate cancer is between 10% and 15%, and the average man's risk of dying from prostate cancer is 3%. If other members of your family have had the disease, however, the risk of developing it, and developing it earlier, goes up. If one family member has had prostate cancer, for example, your risk is doubled. If two family members have had prostate cancer, the risk becomes two to five times higher. It doesn't matter whether the person with prostate cancer comes from your mother's or your father's side of the family—the risk is still the same. We think it is more important if it is your primary relative, like your father or brother, but we aren't sure.

Geographic location

Where you live can affect your chances of dying from advanced prostate cancer. Currently, in the United States, about 25% of the men diagnosed with prostate cancer will actually die of it. In Japan, there is a smaller risk of being diagnosed with

Cancer Incidence		Cancer Mortality	
Men		**Men**	
Prostate	43%	Lung	32%
Lung	12%	Prostate	14%
Colon & Rectum	8.5%	Colon & Rectum	9%
Bladder	5%	Pancreas	4.5%
Non-Hodgkin's Lymphoma	4%	Non-Hodgkin's Lymphoma	4%
Melanoma (skin cancer)	3%	Leukemia	4%
Oral Cavity (mouth & throat)	3%	Esophagus	3%
Kidney	2%	Stomach	3%
Leukemia	2%	Bladder	2.5%
Stomach	2%	Liver	2.5%

prostate cancer, but about 33% of the men who are diagnosed with it will die from it. Men in Switzerland who have been diagnosed with prostate cancer have the greatest chance of dying from it—about 30-40% of those diagnosed! The reasons for such variations are not clear, but the possibilities range from genetic causes to diet, to later diagnosis of the disease.

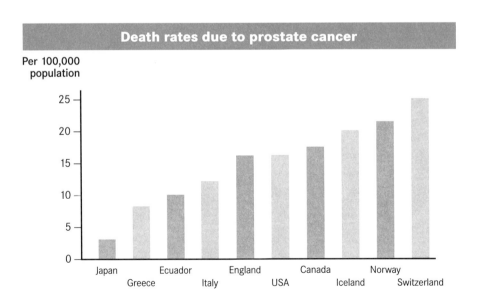

Race

Ethnic background plays a definite role in prostate-cancer risk. Within the United States itself, African-Americans are more likely to die of prostate cancer than members of any other race. As with geographic location, the reasons for these differences are not yet understood.

	African-American	Japanese	Caucasian
Lifetime risk of prostate cancer diagnosis	9%	4 – 5%	13%
Lifetime risk of dying from prostate cancer	4.5%	1%	3.5%

Hormone levels

There is still a lot of work to be done in understanding the relationship between hormones and prostate cancer, but we think that high levels of testosterone are associated with an increased risk of prostate cancer, and low levels of testosterone are associated with a decreased risk of prostate cancer. The picture is more complex than that, however, and may involve other hormones and even enzymes that can change one hormone into another hormone.

For example, men with higher levels of the hormone estradiol, a type of estrogen usually found in larger amounts in women, seem to be at a decreased risk for developing prostate cancer. Also, men with lower levels of Sex-Hormone-Binding Globulin (SHBG), a protein in the bloodstream that binds to testosterone and other hormones, seem to be at an increased risk for prostate cancer. And high levels of something called "Insulin-like Growth Factor," or IGF-1, may be a new marker that can identify those individuals who are at high risk of prostate cancer.

Preventable Risk Factors

Screening

Every man between the ages of 50 and 70 should be screened for prostate cancer with a yearly digital rectal exam and PSA blood test. This should start at age 40 if there is a family history or for African-Americans. It has recently been demonstrated that screening leads to the detection of more cancers that are localized inside of the prostate. This should decrease the number of deaths from advanced

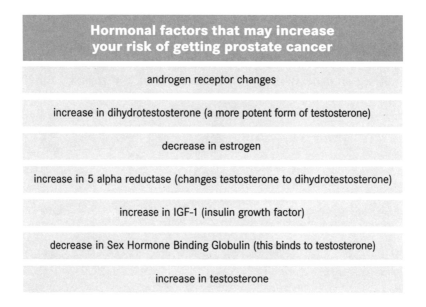

Hormonal factors that may increase your risk of getting prostate cancer
androgen receptor changes
increase in dihydrotestosterone (a more potent form of testosterone)
decrease in estrogen
increase in 5 alpha reductase (changes testosterone to dihydrotestosterone)
increase in IGF-1 (insulin growth factor)
decrease in Sex Hormone Binding Globulin (this binds to testosterone)
increase in testosterone

prostate cancer as more and more men are cured by primary treatments such as surgery or radiation. Lack of screening increases the chance of being diagnosed with advanced disease.

Environment

While race and location play a role in prostate cancer, when men move from one country to another, they eventually come close to achieving the prostate-cancer risk of their adopted nation. So, if a Chinese man moves from China—where only a small number of men die of prostate cancer—to the United States, his risk of dying from prostate cancer increases to become comparable to that of the average American male.

This is another area that is not well understood, but a variety of clues are emerging. Some scientists suspect that exposure to the sun has an effect on the disease. In the United States, for example, men living in the South have a smaller chance of dying from prostate cancer than men living in the North. The theory is that exposure to ultraviolet (UV) radiation from the sun has a protective effect against prostate cancer—perhaps because UV activates the production of vitamin D in the body, which has been known to have some anticancer effects. This may help explain why prostate cancer death rates are highest in areas with less exposure to the sun's rays, such as Scandinavia and North America. This sun-exposure theory also may help explain why African-American men—even those who live in southern climates—are about twice as likely to develop prostate cancer as anyone else, since their highly pigmented skin absorbs less UV. In addition, this theory may also partially explain why older men of any race are at a higher risk of developing prostate cancer, because as we age, our body's ability to make vitamin D from the sun decreases.

Diet

A diet high in saturated fat (especially animal fat) and low in fiber may increase the risk of prostate cancer. Studies have shown that prostate tumors grow faster in animals fed a high-fat diet. People who live in Asia tend to eat less fat than Americans, which may be a partial explanation for the lower incidence of death from prostate cancer in China and Japan. Beans, lentils, green peas, and even strawberries have been identified by some as being helpful in lowering risk; however, the strongest data appear to support a balanced diet low in fat and high in fiber, vegetables, and fruit.

Occupation

Jobs in a number of fields—such as water treatment, aircraft manufacturing, railway transport, utilities, farming, fishing, and forestry—have been associated with prostate cancer risk, but the evidence so far suggests only a slight or possible association. For every study that suggests an increased risk based on a certain occupation, there seems to be another that suggests that this risk does not exist. Slight risks may be related to occupationally oriented exposure to substances, such as a farmer's use of pesticides. It has been suggested that soldiers exposed to Agent Orange may have an increased risk of getting prostate cancer.

Other Possible Factors

There are a number of other factors that may or may not play a role in prostate cancer, or that have been suspected as playing a role, that you might want to know about. These are discussed below.

Alcohol

A number of studies seem to indicate there is little to no risk of getting prostate cancer due to the consumption of alcohol. Some research has suggested that men who drink heavily have a slightly increased risk—with "heavy drinking" meaning 22 to 60 drinks a week or more over many years. On the other hand, another recent study showed that men consuming 57 drinks or more per week did not have an increased risk of prostate cancer. In any case, men who regularly drink that much are likely to have other health problems that are more pressing than prostate cancer. When it comes to alcohol and prostate cancer, the old saying holds true:"Everything in moderation."A glass of wine or a beer at night probably won't increase your risk of getting prostate cancer.

Biopsy, TURP, or other procedures

A common question that we have been hearing for years is,"Does a biopsy or any other procedure increase my chances of cancer cells going into the bloodstream and spreading beyond the prostate?" Researchers have not agreed on whether a biopsy or TURP (transurethral resection of the prostate, a treatment for benign prostate problems) can spread cancer. Overall, it appears that there is a minimal risk with these procedures, in large part because any cells released into the bloodstream are subject to high pressures and the body's immune cells, which can be very effective at destroying a few stray cancer cells. More important, a biopsy is still the most accurate way of determining whether or not you have cancer and how aggressive your cancer is—it is far better to perform the procedure than to simply "guess" about the presence and aggressiveness of cancer based on lab tests and other indirect clinical information.

If you have to have multiple biopsies for any reason, it may be a good idea to wait several weeks before the next one—which is usually the way such tests are handled. In general, of course, a biopsy should only be done when the presence of cancer is suspected based on other information (such as a physical exam or PSA test). A TURP should only be done on those patients whose noncancerous problems are not treatable by less invasive means such as natural therapy and medication.

PIN (Prostatic Intraepithelial Neoplasia)

PIN is a kind of tissue that is not normal, but is also not cancerous. (The term has replaced the words "dysplasia," "malignant transformation," and "intraductal carcinoma," which you may have heard before.) Many doctors believe that PIN can go on to, or become associated with prostate cancer.

There are two types of PIN: Low-grade PIN, which used to be called "PIN1," and high-grade PIN, which used to be known as "PIN2" or "PIN3." Only high-grade PIN is associated with an increased possibility of having cancer. The discovery of low-grade PIN does not put you at a higher risk of having prostate cancer, and clinicians cannot agree on exactly what it looks like. So, many pathologists have stopped trying to identify and report low-grade PIN. Therefore, when the term "PIN" is used today, it usually means high-grade PIN.

The important things you need to know about PIN are:

► The only way to detect it is by having a biopsy. (The same is true of prostate cancer, by the way.)

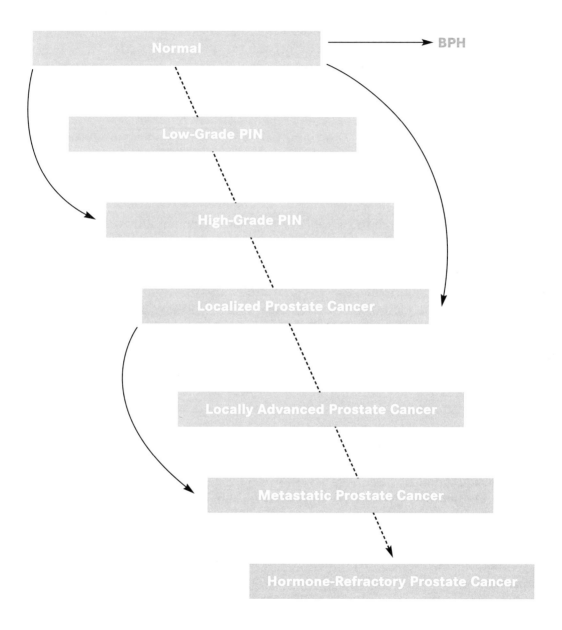

Normal → BPH

Low-Grade PIN

High-Grade PIN

Localized Prostate Cancer

Locally Advanced Prostate Cancer

Metastatic Prostate Cancer

Hormone-Refractory Prostate Cancer

▶ It does not change your PSA to any significant degree.

▶ It usually exists together with prostate cancer. Anywhere from 5% to 40% of the men with prostate cancer also have PIN.

▶ PIN increases with age and may be found up to five years before cancer. The mean age of men with PIN only is 65, compared to a mean age of 70 for men with prostate cancer.

▶ PIN is more common in African-American men than in Caucasian men. It also seems to begin about 10 years earlier in African-Americans.

▶ If you have high-grade PIN on your first biopsy, there is about a 50% chance of being diagnosed with prostate cancer on your next biopsy. The best thing to do if you have been diagnosed with high-grade PIN is to have a repeat biopsy that includes tissue samples from both sides of the prostate, because cancer can occur away from the PIN area.

▶ There is a decrease in the number of cases and amount of PIN with hormonal therapy.

AAH (Atypical Adenomatous Hyperplasia)

These are slightly abnormal cells that usually appear with BPH ("benign prostatic hyperplasia," or enlarged prostate) in an area of the prostate where few prostate cancers are found. AAH can look like cancer to a pathologist, but a test that looks for a "basal layer" can determine whether the cells are AAH or cancer. (The basal layer is disrupted or absent in cancer.) No one is sure whether AAH puts you at an increased risk of having prostate cancer.

Smoking

Numerous studies indicate either a slight prostate cancer risk or no risk at all for men who smoke. Some recent studies suggest a possible increase in the risk of dying from prostate cancer if the man continues to smoke after diagnosis. One thing we do know—smoking doesn't decrease your risk of getting prostate cancer, and it definitely increases your risk of lung cancer. So quitting—or not starting—is a good idea in any case.

Vasectomy

A few years ago, the National Institutes of Health (NIH) reviewed all the information concerning vasectomy and prostate cancer and found no relationship. Therefore, a vasectomy has not been determined to be a risk factor for prostate cancer, and it probably does not decrease your risk either.

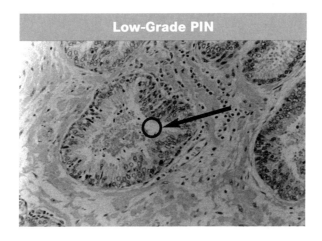

Low-Grade PIN

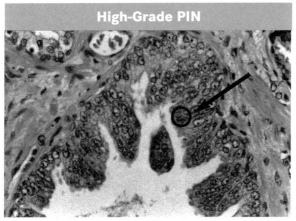

High-Grade PIN

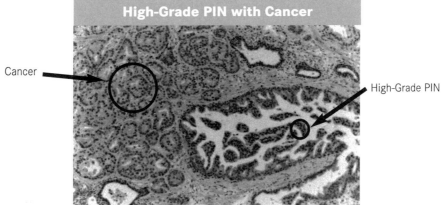

High-Grade PIN with Cancer

Cancer

High-Grade PIN

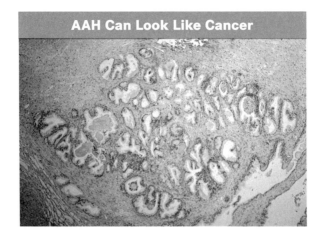

AAH Can Look Like Cancer

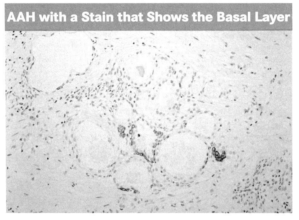

AAH with a Stain that Shows the Basal Layer

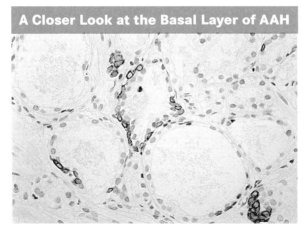

A Closer Look at the Basal Layer of AAH

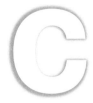

How Can I Tell If I Have Advanced Prostate Cancer? What Are the Symptoms?

Prostate cancer that is confined to the prostate displays few, if any, symptoms. There are some symptoms of general, noncancerous prostate problems that sometimes also appear with prostate cancer—usually, some form of difficulty with the bladder and urinating. But it's important to remember that the presence of these symptoms does not mean you have cancer. In fact, such symptoms are more common to enlarged prostate, (BPH, benign prostate hyperplasia or benign prostatic hypertrophy) or to inflammation of the prostate (prostatitis, which is usually caused by an infection). Basically, there are no urinary symptoms that can be used to definitively diagnose cancer of the prostate. As we mentioned earlier, the only way to truly diagnose prostate cancer is through a biopsy.

If the prostate cancer advances to the seminal vesicles, it can lead to blood in the seminal fluid and/or a decrease in the amount of seminal fluid that is released after ejaculation. If the cancer advances to the nerve bundles around the prostate, the man may experience impotence. And if cancer has spread to the bones, the man may experience bone or back pain and fatigue. Once again, however, it's important to remember that these symptoms are not specific to prostate cancer.

So, if you have prostate cancer, it is likely that you won't have any symptoms, and if you are experiencing symptoms, such as difficulties with urination, they may well be caused by other conditions. The rule here is to have regular prostate checkups and have any urinary difficulty treated by a physician, who will probably perform a digital rectal exam, conduct a PSA test, or, in some situations, perform a transrectal ultrasound to find the source of the problem.

Symptoms of Prostate Cancer

Localized prostate cancer	Advanced or widespread metastatic prostate cancer
Most often no symptoms	Maybe no symptoms* Bone pain Difficulty in urinating Fatigue Weight loss

Locally advanced prostate cancer	
Most often no symptoms	

Regionally advanced prostate cancer	
Most often no symptoms	*Note: About 90% (9 out of 10) of the men diagnosed with advanced prostate cancer have no symptoms.

Quick Review

A. What Should I Know about Prostate Cancer and Advanced Prostate Cancer?

Prostate cancer is an increasingly common disease that affects 1 in 8 men. It is a serious disease that kills some 40,000 men a year. These deaths are due to advanced prostate cancer—that is, cancer that has spread beyond the prostate gland. Conservative estimates indicate that 40% or more of men with prostate cancer will develop some type of advanced cancer.

B. How Does Prostate Cancer Become Advanced?

Advanced prostate cancer is essentially localized prostate cancer that has spread after treatment has failed or because the cancer was not diagnosed in the localized stages. No one really knows what causes prostate cancer, but there are certain factors that increase your risk of getting the disease. Some of these factors, such as screening, are under your control. Others, such as family history and age, are not.

C. How Can I Tell If I Have Advanced Prostate Cancer? What Are the Symptoms?

A person with prostate cancer may have no symptoms. Or, they may have symptoms, such as urinary problems, that are also associated with diseases other than cancer. In some cases, if the cancer has spread beyond the prostate, it may lead to impotence, blood in the seminal fluid, or pain. Because it is difficult to identify prostate cancer on the basis of symptoms alone, check with your doctor if you have any concerns.

2

An Absolutely
Essential Review:
Anatomy and
Function of the
Prostate and
Related Structures

In this chapter:

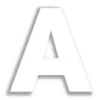

What Do I Need to Know about the Anatomy of the Prostate?

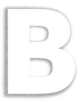

What Do I Need to Know about the Areas near the Prostate?

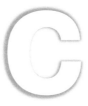

What Do I Need to Know about the Rest of the Body?

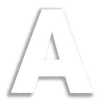

What Do I Need To Know about The Anatomy of the Prostate?

As early as 335 B.C., people knew that the prostate was deep in the body, just below the bladder and above the rectum—and that's about all they knew. Today, we know a lot more, and we're going to summarize some of it in this chapter.

You have probably heard some of this information before, but we think it's worth reviewing. If you have advanced prostate cancer, you will have to deal with a lot of medical jargon and make a lot of decisions, and some basic knowledge of prostate physiology and anatomy will help you understand and participate in your treatment.

In particular, this information will empower you to get the most out of the time you spend with your doctor. Many aspects of your case are specific to you and your situation, from the nature of your disease to the specialties and strengths of various hospitals in your area. This means that a dialogue with your doctor is a critical part of your treatment—and the information in this chapter will help make that dialogue clear and productive.

So let's begin our review.

The Zones of the Prostate

The adult prostate is made up of three major zones. (Other zones exist, but they are very small and do not play a significant role in prostate cancer.).

The peripheral zone

The largest of the three, the peripheral zone makes up about two-thirds of the prostate. It encompasses the back and sides of the gland, from the bottom (also called the "apex") almost all the way to the top (also called the "base"). That may sound upside down, but the bottom of the prostate has more of a pointed end, hence the name "apex," while the top of the prostate is wide and flat and sits below the bladder—hence the name "base."

Front view of the Peripheral Zone (PZ) of the Prostate

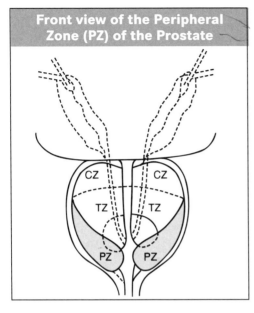

Side view of the Peripheral Zone (PZ) of the Prostate

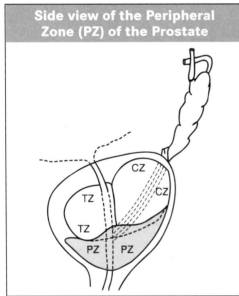

This zone comprises 65-70% of the total area of the prostate (the largest zone of the prostate). 70% of the cancers begin here. Most biopsy samples are taken from here.

When a physician inserts an index finger into the rectum to conduct a Digital Rectal Exam, or DRE, he or she can only feel the peripheral zone. The good news is that this is where the majority of prostate cancers begin. The bad news is that prostate cancers can also begin in the other two zones, which cannot be reached with the index finger.

The central zone

This second-largest zone is a cone-shaped region that makes up the majority of the base and much of the central portion of the prostate. It surrounds the ejaculatory ducts, where sperm from the testicles and fluid from the seminal vesicles meet to flow into the urethra. About 5% to 10% of prostate cancers begin growing in this zone which, as we said, cannot be examined with a DRE.

The transition zone

This is the smallest of the three zones: It is made up of two equal-sized lobes, one on each side of the prostatic urethra. We sometimes call this the BPH zone, because benign prostate hyperplasia, or noncancerous enlargement of the prostate, occurs only in this zone. Since this zone surrounds the urethra, BPH can cause many problems with urinary flow. About 15% to 20% of prostate cancers begin in the transition zone, which of course cannot be reached by DRE. However, since a number of cancers begin growing here, some physicians take biopsies from this area, as well as from the peripheral zone.

The Prostatic Capsule

The prostatic capsule is the outer portion of the prostate. The capsule is significant in advanced disease because if it has been penetrated by cancer, there is a greater possibility that the disease has or will spread beyond the prostate. If the capsule does not have signs of cancer, there's a good chance that the disease is still confined to the prostate.

Surgical Margins

When a surgeon cuts around the prostate during a radical prostatectomy, the prostate and the areas removed with it are sent to a pathologist for examination. The pathologist looks at the outer edges of this sample—the margins—to see if there is cancer present. If there is, there is a greater chance that the cancer has spread beyond the area removed during surgery. If those margins do not contain cancer, there is a greater possibility that the cancer is confined to the prostate. Therefore, you may hear that your prostate is margin positive (+) after surgery, meaning that some cancer was found there, or you may hear that your prostate is margin negative (-), which means no cancer was found there.

This zone comprises 20-25% of the total area of the prostate (the second largest zone of the prostate). 5-10% of the cancers begin here. A DRE cannot feel this area and a biopsy sample is usually not taken from here.

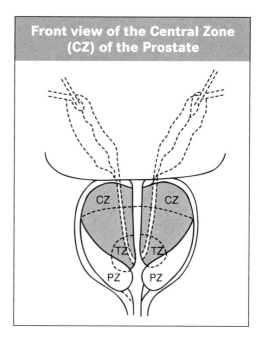

Front view of the Central Zone (CZ) of the Prostate

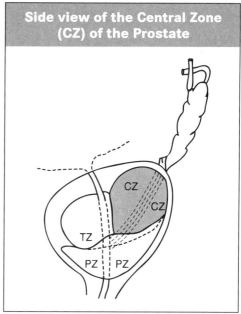

Side view of the Central Zone (CZ) of the Prostate

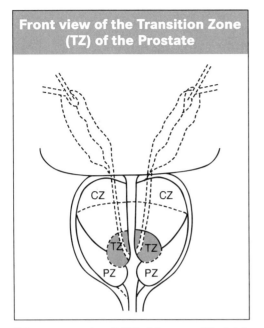

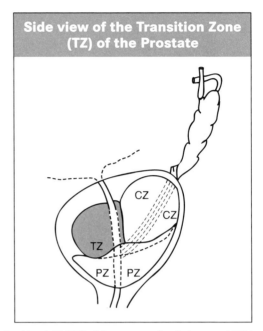

This zone comprises 5-10% of the area of the total prostate. About 15-20% of the cancers begin here and BPH occurs here. A DRE cannot feel this area, but sometimes part of the biopsy sample is taken from here.

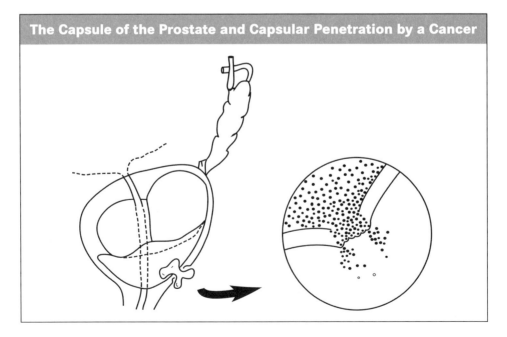

Apical Margin and Basilar or Bladder Neck Margin

The apical margin is the part of the capsule near the bottom of the prostate, close to the urethra where it leaves the prostate. (It's near the apex, mentioned earlier, which is why it's called "apical"). The basilar or bladder neck margin is the part of the capsule that's close to the top of the prostate and near the bladder.

It is important to know about these two areas because if cancer is found in the apical margin after a radical prostatectomy, it may not be very significant—in other words, it does not necessarily mean that the cancer will move to adjacent areas. However, if there is cancer in the basilar or bladder neck margin, there is an increased possibility that the cancer has spread outside of the prostate.

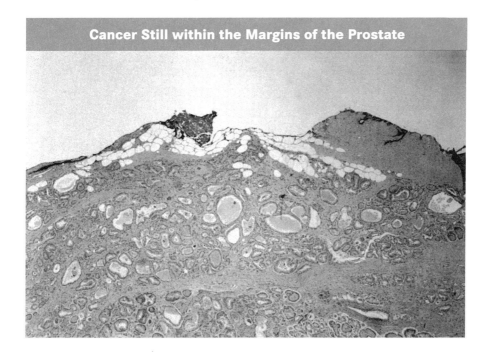

Cancer Still within the Margins of the Prostate

A Closer Look at a Cancer Still within the Margins of the Prostate

Margins

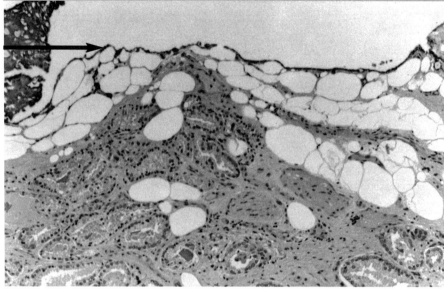

Cancer That Has Spread outside the Margins of the Prostate

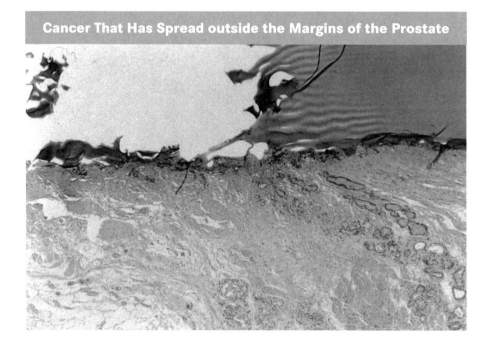

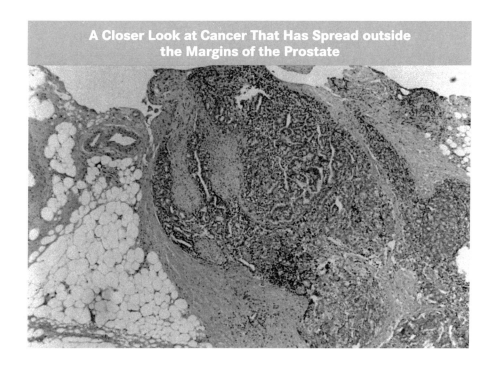

A Closer Look at Cancer That Has Spread outside the Margins of the Prostate

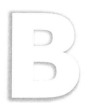

What Do I Need To Know about the Areas near the Prostate?

Neurovascular Bundles and Perineural Invasion

The neurovascular bundles are lengths of nerves, one on the left side of the prostate and one on the right, located near the rectum. These nerve bundles are very tiny, and difficult to find with the naked eye. Each carries nerves and blood to the penis to assist in achieving an erection. A few years ago, when we did not know these bundles existed, a radical prostatectomy often damaged them, causing most patients to become impotent. Even if one or both of the bundles is

The Dorsal Vein Complex of the Prostate

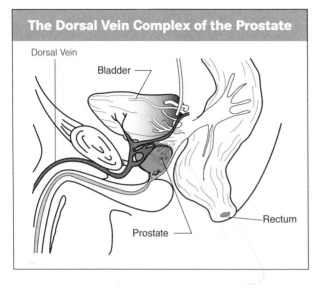

Dorsal Vein

Bladder

Rectum

Prostate

spared during surgery, it does not guarantee that the patient will be able to have natural erections—but it does increase the probability that he will, especially if he is younger. In some cases, the doctor may not be able to spare these nerve bundles because they have cancer or because they may allow the cancer easier access to other parts of the body. It all depends on where the cancer is located at the time of surgery. Your doctor may use the term "perineural invasion," which means that the cancer has invaded one or both nerve bundles or the area around them.

Dorsal Vein Complex

Blood is drained from the prostate by a number of veins which together are called the "dorsal vein complex." When removing the prostate, surgeons have to be careful not to nick these veins because they carry a large amount of blood.

Seminal Vesicles

The seminal vesicles play a large role in advanced prostate cancer. There are two seminal vesicles located behind the bladder that drain into the urethra inside the prostate. Prostate cancer will often spread to the seminal vesicles, so they are typically removed during prostate surgery.

The seminal vesicles make seminal fluid, which mixes with sperm from the testicles to make "semen"—the substance that is released from the penis during ejaculation. After prostate surgery, a man usually has "dry" orgasms because of the removal of the seminal vesicles.

Testicles and Vas Deferens

The testicles make sperm cells, which are transported by tubes (one from each testicle) that drain into the urethra. The ends of these tubes are called the "vas deferens," and these join the seminal vesicles, allowing the sperm and the seminal fluid to mix. The vas deferens lie close to the prostate and are vulnerable to

Where Does Semen Come from and What Is in It?

Semen is sperm plus seminal fluid. Normal semen color is white and a normal sperm count is 100 million sperm cells per millimeter of semen. Testicles make sperm cells. The seminal vesicles make 60% of the seminal fluid and are a common place where cancer can go (they are removed during surgery).

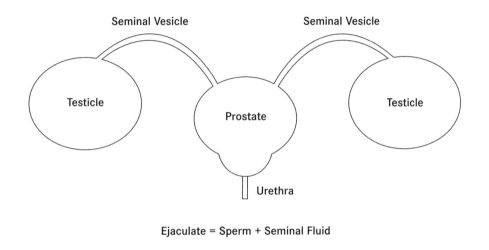

Ejaculate = Sperm + Seminal Fluid

spreading cancer, so both vas deferens are removed during surgery. This is why most men cannot have children after a radical prostatectomy. However, there are techniques that doctors can use to extract sperm from the testicles if a couple wants to have a baby after prostate surgery.

The vas deferens are the part of the anatomy that is cut and clamped when a man has a vasectomy. However, in both prostate surgery and a vasectomy, the doctor is not removing the source of the sperm, just the path it takes. Sometimes, small amounts of sperm will still find their way to the urethra. This only happens in a very small number of cases, but it means that a vasectomy or prostate surgery cannot provide a 100% guarantee that a man will never have a baby naturally again.

The Urethra, the Bladder, and the Ureters

The urethra carries both sperm and urine to the tip of the penis. It begins at the bottom of the bladder and goes through the prostate at an angle, and then leaves the prostate and travels to and through the penis. The bladder stores urine until you urinate, eventually releasing it into the urethra. The urine comes to the bladder from the kidneys by two tubes—the ureters. The bladder is especially significant in prostate cancer, because cancer can spread there.

The Internal and External Sphincter

A sphincter acts as a kind of door, opening and closing a part of the body. The area around the prostate has two sphincters of importance. First, there is the internal sphincter, which is located at the bottom of the bladder next to the point where the urethra begins. This internal sphincter is under "involuntary control," meaning that when the bladder is full, it may open without your thinking about it. The internal sphincter also closes automatically when you have an orgasm so that urine from the bladder does not mix with sperm from the testicles.

The external sphincter is located at the bottom or apex of the prostate where the urethra leaves the prostate. This sphincter is under voluntary control and allows you to hold your urine even if your bladder is ready to be emptied.

During a radical prostatectomy, radiation, or other therapies, the internal sphincter might be partially removed or damaged. In most cases, however, you can still hold your urine with the external sphincter. However, both of these sites can be invaded by cancer from the prostate, and may have to be removed. Cancer can also damage these sphincters. As result, some men who have had prostate treatment or who have advanced prostate cancer suffer from incontinence, or the lack of urinary control. There are techniques that can be used to control incontinence, such as having an artificial sphincter put in or having collagen injections at the site of the internal sphincter.

Denonvilliers' Fascia

Named for Charles Pierre Denonvilliers, the French surgeon who discovered it in the 1800s, Denonvilliers' fascia is a piece of tissue located behind the prostate, separating the prostate from the rectum. Many surgeons remove this fascia when they are doing a radical prostatectomy, because it is an area often invaded by prostate cancer.

Lymph Nodes

The body has a complex network of lymph vessels that transport protein, fat, excess fluid, and other materials. At various points along these vessels are pea-sized lymph nodes, which contain disease-fighting cells. Normally, these nodes are small, but if the body is fighting an infection, they can become enlarged—which is why a doctor might feel the nodes in your neck if you have a sore throat.

There are lymph nodes near the prostate, but they cannot be felt with a finger because they lie deep inside the body. However, they can be seen during surgery or with an imaging test. If cancer cells are present in the prostate area, these nodes may get larger as they fight the disease. In general, the greater the amount of cancer in the node, the larger the node may become. That simple fact provides the basis of part of a prostate cancer staging system, which uses lymph nodes to gauge the seriousness of the cancer. (Staging is discussed in more detail in the next chapter.)

During prostate surgery, tissue from these nodes can be removed and then examined by a pathologist to determine whether or not the cancer has spread. Therefore, you may hear the terms "node positive" (+), meaning cancer was found in the nodes, or node negative (-), meaning no cancer was found. Sometimes, doctors may also refer to the number of nodes affected by cancer, saying "2 out of 10," or "1 out of 4," etc. The larger the number of nodes affected, the more the cancer has spread.

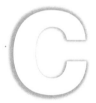

What Do I Need to Know about the Rest of the Body?

Bones, Liver, Lungs, etc.

Cancer that spreads beyond the prostate, seminal vesicles, or local lymph nodes can move to the bones—such as the spine or legs—and organs such as the lungs or the liver. When prostate cancer has spread to these areas, it is much more serious because it is beginning to invade vital parts of the body.

Hormones

Hormones are substances produced by one part of the body that travel in the bloodstream to affect other parts of the body. In men, the primary hormone is testosterone, which plays a role in everything from the production of sperm to the growth or loss of hair (it's also what contributes to balding in some men).

Understanding how testosterone is made in the body will help you understand the hormonal therapy used to treat advanced prostate cancer. In the brain, there is a structure called the hypothalamus that makes a hormone called "Luteinizing

Hormone Releasing Hormone" (LHRH). LHRH travels from the hypothalamus to the anterior pituitary, which is also in the brain, to create "Luteinizing Hormone" (LH). This LH then travels down to the testicles, where it causes cells to make testosterone.

Many prostate cancer cells need testosterone to grow, so doctors use hormonal therapy analogs to try to stop the production of testosterone. This involves regular injections of LHRH, which causes the body to "think" that there is too much LHRH in the system, and to become desensitized to the hormone. In essence, this means that the body begins to ignore the LHRH; the anterior pituitary no longer recognizes it, and so it stops releasing LH, which in turn causes the testicles to stop making testosterone. (When a course of LHRH injections begins, there is actually a large initial increase in testosterone production, but after about two weeks, desensitization takes effect and the testosterone production drops.)

Another approach is to stop the production of testosterone by removing the testicles, a procedure known as "orchiectomy" or "surgical castration." When the testicles are removed, the production of testosterone stops almost immediately— or at least most of it does. About 5% to 10% of the body's testosterone is actually made in the adrenal glands, located on the top of the kidneys.

Cells: Normal, benign, cancer, and so forth....

The human body is made up of some one trillion cells of various kinds. Normal cells perform vital functions in the body and, when grouped with other similar cells, make up an organ or a tissue.

Benign cells are cells that are abnormal, but not cancerous. For example, in Benign Prostatic Hyperplasia, or BPH, the prostate becomes abnormally large because the prostate cells begin acting abnormally, making more than the normal number of cells. Some benign cells may change into cancerous cells over time, but this is not believed to be the case with BPH.

Cancer cells of the prostate are different from normal or benign cells, and come in several types. As we mentioned earlier, some cancers cells rely on the presence of testosterone to grow and thrive; these are called "hormone dependent" or "hormone sensitive" cancer cells. These cells can be controlled fairly well with hormone therapy that limits testosterone production. But there are other prostate cancer cells that do not depend on testosterone or other hormones at all. These are called "hormone independent" or "hormone insensitive" cancer cells, and as you might expect, they cannot be managed through hormone therapy.

There are other methods for dealing with hormone-independent cells. Many respond to radiation, but others do not. Chemotherapy and other treatments, which are discussed in more detail later in this book, can also be effective.

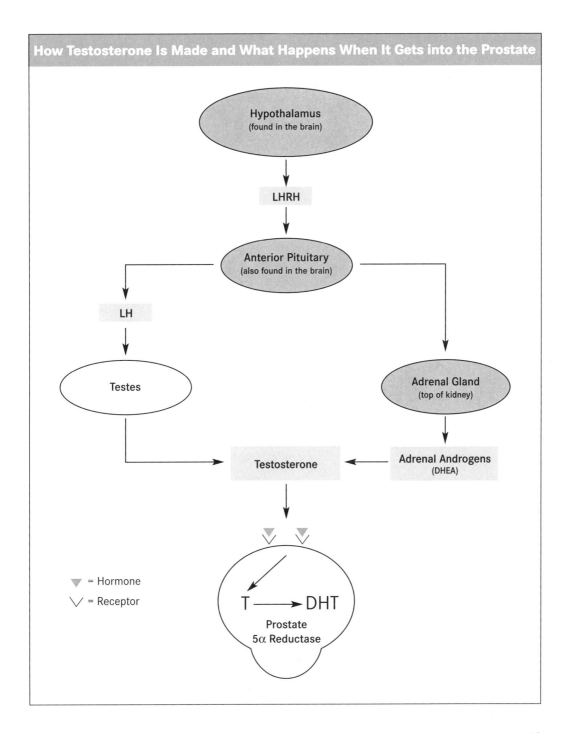

How Testosterone Is Made and What Happens When It Gets into the Prostate

Hypothalamus
(found in the brain)

LHRH

Anterior Pituitary
(also found in the brain)

LH

Testes

Adrenal Gland
(top of kidney)

Testosterone ← Adrenal Androgens
(DHEA)

▼ = Hormone
∨ = Receptor

T ⟶ DHT
Prostate
5α Reductase

So overall, there is quite an arsenal that we can throw at these cancer cells, but there are complications as well. Over time, cancer cells may change to become hormone independent, radiation resistant, or drug resistant. The good news is that researchers are continually exploring new ways to kill cancer cells. You will read about many of these discoveries later in this book.

Quick Review

A. What Do I Need To Know about the Anatomy of the Prostate?
The prostate gland has three major zones: the peripheral zone, the central zone, and the transition zone. Cancer is most likely to occur in the peripheral zone—which is by far the largest of the three—but it can occur in the other zones as well.

The areas and structures on and around the outer boundary of the prostate play an important role in assessing prostate cancer, because doctors can examine these margins and edges to determine whether cancer has started to spread beyond the prostate.

B. What Do I Need to Know about the Areas near the Prostate?
There are a number of complex and delicate structures in the area around the prostate. These can be damaged by prostate cancer that spreads beyond the capsule, or by treatment for the cancer itself. In some cases, this damage can result in problems with urinary control and/or impotence. There are techniques that can help in managing some of the side effects.

C. What Do I Need to Know about the Rest of the Body?
Prostate cancer can spread far beyond the immediate area of the prostate to organs and bones elsewhere in the body. In addition, hormones manufactured in other areas of the body can affect the growth of prostate cancer, so doctors sometimes try to control hormone production to control cancer.

Finally, just as there are many kinds of cells in the body, there can also be various types of cancer cells. Some of these cancer cells respond to hormone therapy, some to radiation, and some to drugs, so treatments can vary depending on the specific nature of an individual's disease.

3

Another Absolutely Essential Review: Grading and Staging Your Cancer

In this chapter:

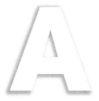

What Do I Need to Know about the Grading Systems?

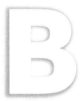

What Do I Need to Know about the ABCD and TNM Staging Systems?

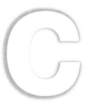

What Is the Difference between Localized, Locally Advanced, Regionally Advanced, and Advanced or Metastatic Prostate Cancer?

In Chapter 2, we looked at the basics of anatomy and physiology. Now, we need to review some information about prostate cancer, such as how it is assessed, and how it can advance. Once again, some of this may be information you already know, but we think it's worth reviewing in order to arm you with the knowledge you need to be an effective partner in your treatment.

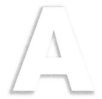

What Do I Need to Know about The Grading Systems?

When you have a prostate cancer biopsy, a sample of tissue is sent to a pathologist to be "graded" or examined in order to understand just how aggressive and fast-growing it might be.

Grading System	Well differentiated or not aggressive	Moderately differentiated or moderately aggressive	Poorly differentiated or very aggressive
Gleason (most popular grading system)	2-4	5-7	8-10
Mostofi (World Health Org.) (second most popular grading system)	I	II	III
Broders and M.D. Anderson Cancer Center	1-2	2-3	4

There are many grading systems used by doctors. These systems vary, of course, but they are all designed to give you and your doctor some insight into the nature of the cancer by categorizing it with a grade. The higher the grade, the more the cancer cells do not look like normal cells—and therefore, the more aggressive the cancer and the more likely it is that it will grow and spread quickly. Conversely, the lower the grade, the more your cancer cells look like normal cells—and therefore, the less aggressive the cancer and the more likely it is that the disease will grow and spread slowly.

The most widely used grading system is the Gleason Grading System. To come up with a Gleason grade, a pathologist looks at the cancer tissue and assigns it two numbers between 1 and 5. Two numbers are given because prostate tumors from a single individual will usually show some variation. In other words, some of the tumor might look aggressive, while some of it may not. The pathologist is concerned about the overall appearance of the tumor, and so uses the grades of the two most predominant types of tissue, and combines them to come up with a total score for the tumor. The first number is the most predominant type and the second number is the second most common type seen on the slides.

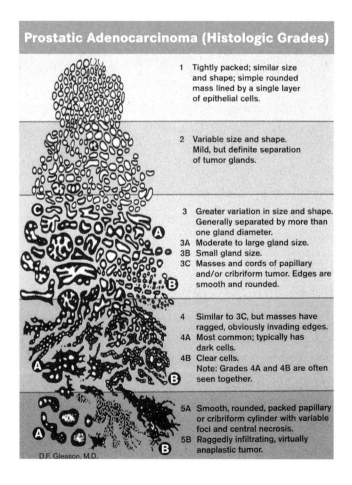

Prostatic Adenocarcinoma (Histologic Grades)

1 Tightly packed; similar size and shape; simple rounded mass lined by a single layer of epithelial cells.

2 Variable size and shape. Mild, but definite separation of tumor glands.

3 Greater variation in size and shape. Generally separated by more than one gland diameter.
3A Moderate to large gland size.
3B Small gland size.
3C Masses and cords of papillary and/or cribriform tumor. Edges are smooth and rounded.

4 Similar to 3C, but masses have ragged, obviously invading edges.
4A Most common; typically has dark cells.
4B Clear cells.
Note: Grades 4A and 4B are often seen together.

5A Smooth, rounded, packed papillary or cribriform cylinder with variable foci and central necrosis.
5B Raggedly infiltrating, virtually anaplastic tumor.

D.F. Gleason. M.D.

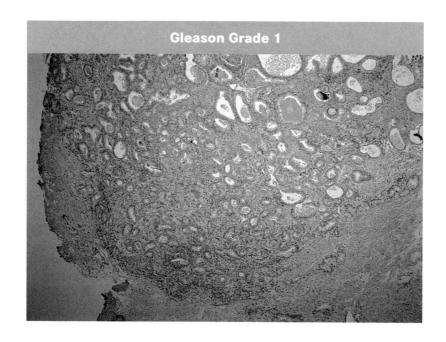

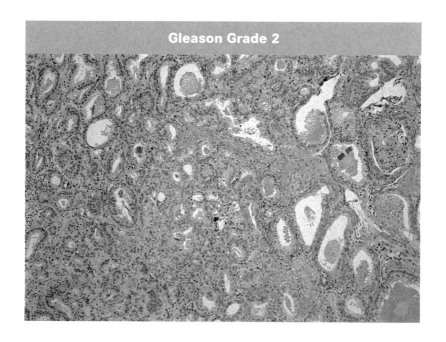

Gleason Grade 3

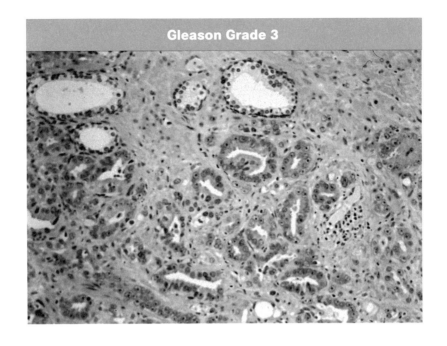

Gleason Grade 4

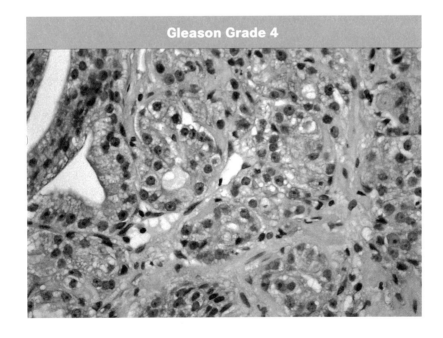

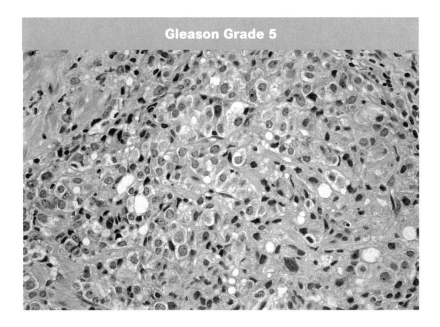

Gleason Grade 5

A Gleason total score will be somewhere between 2 and 10, with scores between 2 and 4 being the least aggressive cancers, 5 through 7 being moderately aggressive, and 8 through 10 being very aggressive. A pathology report might say that a Gleason score is "3+4=7," which tells you the total and the two individual scores used to reach that total. Other reports might just say "3+4," or "7 total" or "7 overall." You should always be sure to ask your doctor for the full set of numbers—the total Gleason score and the two subscores. This is because many doctors are beginning to think that it is only the most predominant type of cancer that is important for prognosis; that is, telling whether your cancer has already or may someday spread. For example, a 3+4=7 may be better to have than a 4+3=7 cancer. (Remember, the first number is the most predominant type and the second number is the second most common type seen on the slides.) However, it is still too early to know for sure if this is true.

It is important to note that the Gleason system has recently undergone a minor change, which has yet to be fully adopted by the medical community. In the newer version, there is a separate category or number (Gleason of 7) for a moderately poorly-aggressive prostate cancer. In the older system, the Gleason of number 7 was grouped with the numbers 5 and 6. This change was made because over the past several years, physicians have noticed that cancers with Gleason scores of 7 do not look or act like those with scores of 5 and 6 or 8 and 10. So they have been given their own category.

Older Gleason System	Newer Gleason System	What does it mean?
2-4	2-4	A well-differentiated cancer that looks a lot like normal prostate cells and is slightly aggressive
5-7	5-6	A moderately-differentiated cancer that looks somewhat like normal cells and is moderately aggressive
—	7	A moderately poorly-differentiated cancer that looks only a little like normal cells and is aggressive
8-10	8-10	A poorly-differentiated cancer that does not look anything like normal cells and is very aggressive

All the possible Gleason scores you can receive	What does that tell us?
1+1, 2+1, 1+2, 1+3 2+1, 2+2 3+1	2-4 = Well differentiated cancer or not aggressive
1+4, 1+5 2+3, 2+4 3+2, 3+3 4+1, 4+2 5+1	5-6 = Moderately differentiated cancer or moderately aggressive
2+5 3+4 4+3 5+2	7 = Moderately poorly-differentiated or aggressive
3+5 4+4, 4+5 5+3, 5+4, 5+5	8-10 = Poorly differentiated cancer or very aggressive

Statistically, here is what we know about total Gleason scores and advanced cancer:

▶ 2.1% of the Gleason scores of 2 - 4 spread beyond the prostate in a year if they are not treated. Therefore, in five years the chances of spread are about 10%; in 10 years, about 20-25%; in 15 years about 30-33%; and in 20 years about 40-45%. That is, of course, fairly slow growth—and not surprisingly, the majority of older men with localized cancer and a low Gleason score die of something other than prostate cancer, regardless of whether they have treatment.

▶ 5.4% of the Gleason scores of 5 - 7 will spread beyond the prostate in a year if they are not treated. Therefore, in five years the chances of spread are about 25-30%; in 10 years, about 50-55%; in 15 years about 80-85%; and in 20 years, about 100%.

▶ 13.5% of the Gleason scores 8 to 10 will spread beyond the prostate in a year if they are not treated. Therefore, in five years the chances of spread are about 65-70%, and in 10 years, about 100%. Clearly, then, men with high Gleason scores have a much higher risk of getting advanced prostate cancer.

Many patients wonder if their Gleason score can change over time. Research seems to indicate that it usually does not change that much—so a 5 today will probably mean a 5 tomorrow. However, doctors may change their minds about what your score is. Different pathologists may disagree on your Gleason score, or the biopsy may have revealed only part of your cancer, making the Gleason number inaccurate. In fact, about 25% of the Gleason scores are "undergraded," meaning the score is lower than it should be for the cancer in question. And about 25% of the Gleason scores are "overgraded," with a number that is higher than it should be.

If you are concerned about your Gleason score, have another pathologist read your biopsy. This may be especially appropriate for lower-to-moderate Gleason scores because these are more likely to be inaccurate. High Gleason scores mean the cancer looks very different from the normal prostate cells, so such cells are easier to identify. As a result, higher scores tend to be more accurate.

We always stress the importance of knowing your Gleason scores. In fact, we are often surprised at the number of patients who know every PSA number they have ever received, but have no idea of their total Gleason score at the time of initial diagnosis. A Gleason score gives you and your doctor an idea of how aggressive your cancer may be, which helps determine the kind of treatment you may need.

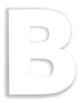

What Do I Need to Know About the ABCD and TNM Staging Systems?

In addition to knowing how aggressive a man's prostate cancer is, doctors also want to determine how far it has spread, and where it is located. Making this determination is called "staging" the cancer.

There are two types of staging systems in use today: The ABCD system (also called the Whitmore-Jewett system), and the newer TNM staging system. Some doctors use one, some use the other, and some use both. Therefore, it is important to understand both systems.

The ABCD system uses those four letters to describe stages:

► "A" means the tumor is localized and was found during a procedure unrelated to cancer, such as a TURP, which is a surgery for the treatment of BPH.

► "B" means the tumor is still localized, but was found by DRE, PSA, or some other method used to detect cancer.

► "C" means the tumor has left the prostate and may have reached other structures near the prostate.

► "D" means the tumor has spread far beyond the prostate to the lymph nodes, lungs, bone, or other organs.

A number from 0 to 2 is usually placed next to the letter. The higher the number, the more space the cancer takes up in that location or the farther it has spread. So, for example, a C2 cancer and a C1 cancer have both left the prostate, as indicated by the letter C, but the C2 has spread farther.

The TNM staging system is more specific about the location of the cancer. It has just recently been updated, so we refer to it as the "new" TNM system. In this system:

► **T** stands for "tumor." When a tumor is staged, the report will include a capital

T with a number between 1 and 4, and a lower-case letter (a, b, or c) next to it. The greater the number and letter, the farther the cancer has spread. For example, a T2b is confined to the prostate but covers more area than a T2a cancer. A T3b cancer has spread a little beyond the prostate, while a T4 cancer has spread far beyond the prostate. If you do not have prostate cancer, then your report may include a capital T with a zero (T0).

▶ **N** stands for "nodes." If the lymph nodes contain cancer, the staging report will include a capital N (for nodes) with a plus sign next to it: "N+," as well as a T. If the lymph nodes do not contain cancer, the report will include a capital N with a zero (N0). An "x" (Nx) is used if the status of the lymph nodes is not known.

▶ **M** stands for "metastasis." If the cancer has spread far beyond the prostate—to the bones, for example—then the staging report will include a capital M. If the cancer has not spread far beyond the prostate, the report may include a

The ABCD and New TNM Clinical Staging Systems for Localized Prostate Cancer		
ABCD	**TNM**	**What do the results mean?**
—	**TX**	The cancer cannot be staged at this time.
—	**TO**	There is no evidence of a cancer.
A	**T1**	A cancer that cannot be felt with a DRE or picked up by an imaging machine (x-ray, CT scan, MRI, etc.) or is found by PSA or another procedure, such as a TURP for BPH. This is "localized or confined prostate cancer."
A1	**T1a**	A cancer that is found during a procedure such as a TURP (not found by a biopsy). The cancer takes up less than 5% of prostate tissue removed in the procedure.
A2	**T1b**	A cancer that is found during a procedure such as a TURP. The cancer takes up more than 5% of the prostate tissue removed in the procedure.
B0	**T1c**	A cancer that cannot be felt with a DRE but it is detected by a biopsy in one or both sides of the prostate, because of an initial high PSA level.
B1 or B2	**T2**	The cancer is only confined or within the prostate, and/or it has invaded the apex of the prostate (where the urethra leaves the prostate), or it has gone into but not beyond the prostate capsule. This is still called a "localized or confined prostate cancer."
B1	**T2a**	A cancer that occupies only one side (lobe) of the prostate.
B2	**T2b**	A cancer that occupies both sides (lobes) of the prostate.

Note: There is no longer a T2c cancer with the newer system.

The ABCD and New TNM Clinical Staging Systems for Advanced Prostate Cancer

ABCD	TNM	What do the results mean?
C1-C2	T3	The cancer goes through the prostate capsule. This is also called "locally advanced prostate disease."
C1	T3a	A cancer on one or both sides of the prostate that is now growing on the outside and going beyond the prostate. This is also called "unilateral (one side) or bilateral (both sides) extracapsular extension."
C2	T3b	A cancer that has invaded one or both seminal vesicles.
		Note: There is no longer a T3c cancer with the newer system.
C2	T4	A cancer that has spread to or invaded other nearby structures other than the seminal vesicle(s) such as the: bladder neck, external sphincter, rectum, nearby muscles (also called "levator muscles") and/or the pelvic wall. This is also called a "locally or regionally advanced prostate cancer."
		Note: There is no longer a T4a or T4b prostate cancer with the newer system.
—	NX	The lymph nodes cannot be staged at this time.
—	N0	No lymph nodes near the prostate have cancer (or metastasis). These are also called "regional lymph nodes."
D1	N1	Cancer in a regional node or nodes near the prostate. This is also called a "regionally advanced prostate cancer."
		Note: There is no longer a N2 or N3 prostate cancer or an N+ cancer with the newer system.
		Also note: The regional lymph nodes are in the pelvic area and there are 5 sets of them called: Pelvic, Hypogastric, Obturator, Iliac, and Sacral.
—	MX	Metastasis or cancer spread far beyond the prostate (also called "distant metastasis") cannot be staged at this time.
—	M0	There is no metastasis or cancer spread far beyond the prostate (also called "no distant metastasis").
D2	M1	Cancer has metastasized or spread far beyond the prostate (also called "distant metastasis"). This is also called an "Advanced Prostate Cancer."
D2	M1a	Cancer has metastasized or spread to a node or nodes far beyond the prostate (also called "nonregional lymph node or nodes").
D2	M1b	Cancer has metastasized or spread to the bone or bones.
D2	M1c	Cancer has metastasized or spread to another site or sites in the body far beyond the prostate (such as the liver, lungs, and bones. This is the most advanced category or stage of prostate cancer.)

ABCD	TNM	What do the results mean?
		Note: The newer staging system has added an M1b and M1c category and has eliminated the M+ category.
		Also note: The nonregional lymph nodes are far from the prostate and there are 8 sets of them called: Aortic (also called "para-aortic lumbar"), Common iliac, Inguinal, Superficial inguinal (also called "femoral"), Supraclavicular, Cervical, Scalene, and Retroperitoneal.
		Also note: M or Metastasis, or cancer spread far beyond the prostate commonly goes to the bone or bones. In addition, during metastasis the cancer can commonly go to nonregional or distant lymph nodes. Prostate cancer to the lung is uncommon with metastasis but when it occurs it usually is because it has gone along the distant lymph nodes to eventually reach the lung. Liver metastasis or cancer that has spread to the liver is very uncommon and it usually occurs late in the course of this disease.

capital M with a zero (M0). An "x"(Mx) is used if it is unknown whether someone has metastatic disease.

Clinical Staging and Pathological Staging

When we talk about staging cancer with systems such as ABCD and TNM, we are usually referring to "clinical staging." That means the staging is based on clinical information, such as a DRE, a PSA, ultrasound tests, etc. Clinical staging is really only an estimate of how far your cancer has spread, and it can never be 100% accurate because we are not looking around inside the body to gather information.

As a result, the stage of cancer can be underestimated or overestimated in clinical staging. For example, doctors may believe that a cancer is T3 based on the clinical information, but in reality it may turn out to be a T2 or relatively confined prostate cancer. In that case, the cancer would have been overestimated or "overstaged." Or, on the other hand, a patient may have been identified as having a clinical stage of T2, but actually turn out to have a T3. Here, the cancer has been "understaged." The problem, of course, is that such inaccuracies can lead to the use of ineffective treatment, or to lost treatment opportunities. As with the grading of cancers discussed above, about 25% of patients have their cancers overstaged, and another 25% or so have them understaged—but in the hands of an experienced physician, your chances of being accurately staged through clinical methods are very good.

The most accurate way to determine how far a cancer has spread is through pathological staging—that is, by actually looking at samples of all the tissue in question. But there's a catch: The only patients who are candidates for pathological staging are those who have had a radical prostatectomy, which provides the pathologist with the tissue to examine.

There is a system created specifically for pathological staging. Known as "pT," this system describes the spread of cancer to areas around the prostate. It does not encompass areas far beyond the prostate, because there are other techniques, such as imaging and biopsies that are used to identify cancer in the bones, lungs, liver etc.

Many patients who have had a biopsy or surgery to remove the prostate keep a copy of their pathology report for their records. We encourage you to do this. This report gives you and your doctor a clear idea of how far the cancer has spread and just how aggressive it is.

The Pathologic Staging System. Also Known as pT

The small p means "pathologic" while the capital T means "Tumor."

Pathologic Stage	What does that really mean?
pT2	This is a localized or prostate (organ) confined cancer.
pT2a	This is a prostate cancer that is localized or confined to only one side of the prostate. It is also called a "unilateral" prostate cancer.
pT2b	This is a prostate cancer that is localized or confined to both sides of the prostate. It is also called a "bilateral" prostate cancer.
pT3	This is a prostate cancer that has spread just beyond the prostate. It is also called "extraprostatic extension."
pT3a	This is a prostate cancer that has barely spread beyond the prostate. It is also called "extraprostatic extension."
pT3b	This is a prostate cancer that has spread to the seminal vesicle(s), which are located near the prostate.
pT4	This is a prostate cancer that has spread to the bladder and/or rectum.
	Note: There is no pathologic T1 category and there is no category beyond T4. For example, there is no pN (for lymph nodes) and there is no pM (for metastatic spread).

An Example Pathological Report from Surgery

(or some of this information can come from the biopsy). Note: Obviously these reports can differ somewhat from hospital to hospital. However, this is some of the standard information it should contain.

Tissue Evalution

Prostate size_____cm x _____cm x _____ (cm=centimeters)

Prostate weight _____g (g=grams)

Seminal vesicles size_____cm x _____cm x _____cm

Seminal vesicles weight_____g

Unilateral cancer? (one side only) Bilateral cancer? (both sides of the prostate)

Pelvic lymphadenectomy tissue submitted? (lymph node samples)

Diagnosis

Radical prostatectomy? Retropubic? Perineal?

Adenocarcinoma (cancer)

Gleason Grade=_____ + _____=_____

Gleason Grade _____ pattern: _____%

Gleason Grade _____ pattern: _____%

Size=_____cc (cc=cubic centimeters)

Location=Unilateral? Bilateral? Peripheral Zone? and/or Transition zone? and/or
   Central Zone?

Surgical or resection margins=Positive? Negative?

Capsule involvement? Within capsule? Beyond capsule (extraprostatic)?
   Unifocal (one-site)? Multifocal (cancer at more than one site)?

Perineural (neurovascular bundle) invasion?

Premalignant change? High-grade PIN?

Pelvic lymph nodes? Cancer? How many nodes are positive?

Prostate Apex? Positive? Negative (for cancer)?

Bladder base? Positive? Negative (for cancer)?

Vascular/lymphatic involvement (invasion)? Yes (extensive or not)? No?

TNM stage? T (Tumor)_____? N (Nodes)_____? M (Metastasis)_____?

Other observations: BPH? Prostatitis?...

Optional (other tests on the samples and results):

Cores (biopsy samples)=Number of cores taken? Number positive (with cancer)?
   Total length of cancer in any core? percent of cancer in each core?...

DNA content (from flow cytometry/ploidy analysis: Diploid? Aneuploid? Tetraploid?

A Second Type of Pathological Report

In this example, the patient has a Gleason score of 4+3=7, with locally advanced disease to 1 seminal vesicle.

Mapping Report

Location	Diagnosis	Core Length(mm)	Tumor Length(mm)	% Tumor	Tumor Position from Inked Margin
Left Apex (Core 1/1)	4+3=7	10	9.0	90%	Not Inked
Left Seminal Vesicle (Core 1/2)	4+3=7	6	6.0	100%	Not Inked
Left Seminal Vesicle (Core 2/2)	4+3=7	8	1.0	12%	Not Inked
Left Mid (Core 1/1)	4+3=7	12	4.0	33%	Not Inked
Right Base (Core 1/1)	4+3=7	15	5.0	33%	Not Inked
Right Mid (Core 1/1)	4+3=7	12	2.0	16%	Not Inked

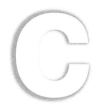

What Is the Difference between Localized, Locally Advanced, Regionally Advanced, and Advanced or Metastatic Prostate Cancer?

The various stages of cancer have been given a number of names, and definitions have changed slightly over the years, so not everyone agrees on the terminology. The term "advanced cancer," used in the title of this book, is a fairly well accepted description of any cancer that is no longer confined to the prostate. However, advanced cancer can actually mean locally advanced, regionally advanced, or advanced/metastatic cancer.

Let's quickly go through some of these terms, and see how they fit with the staging systems described earlier:

▶ **Localized Cancer** is when cancer has not grown beyond the prostate. It is also known as stage T1 or T2 in the TNM system, or stage A or B in the ABCD system.

▶ **Locally Advanced Prostate Cancer** is cancer that has grown just beyond the prostate and/or spread to neighboring tissues, such as the seminal vesicles (stage T3 or C). This also includes cases where the cancer has spread to nearby organs, such as the rectum or bladder (T4 or C). Basically, the term "locally advanced cancer" covers all those cancers that are stage T3 or stage T4, or C.

▶ **Regionally Advanced Cancer** is when cancer has spread to the lymph nodes. This is also known as N1 or D1 prostate cancer.

▶ **Advanced or Metastatic Cancer** is cancer that has spread far beyond the prostate or local lymph nodes to lymph nodes farther from the prostate, or to bones and/or other organs (M1 or D2). However, advanced prostate cancer can also be divided into those cancers that are androgen dependent (also known as "hormone-sensitive") and androgen independent (also known as "hormone-insensitive," "hormone-refractory" or AIPC, which stands for Androgen Independent Prostate Cancer.)

▶ **Recurrence** applies to those cases in which treatment has not been effective. In other words, if after treatment your cancer is not cured or your PSA begins to increase again, then you have experienced a "recurrence." This is not a true cancer stage, but it is useful because it describes a specific situation. Recurring cancer can still be confined to the prostate, or it may have spread to the area around the prostate.

Quick Review

A. What Do I Need to Know about Grading Systems?

A number of grading systems are used to help doctors understand just how aggressive and fast-growing a man's prostate cancer might be. The most common of these is the Gleason grading system, which provides a score of 2 - 10, with the higher numbers corresponding to more-aggressive cancers, and the lower numbers to less-aggressive cancers. The score is produced by totaling two readings from a biopsy. It is important for a man with prostate cancer to know his total Gleason score and the two readings used to create that score.

B. What Do I Need to Know about the ABCD and TNM Staging Systems?

Two systems—ABCD and TNM—are used to stage cancer, or describe how far it has spread from the prostate gland. The TNM is newer and more precise about the location of cancer, but your doctor may use either one of these systems, so it's worth learning about both.

The ABCD and TNM systems are clinical staging systems, which means they are based on clinical observations, such as a DRE or a PSA test. As a result, clinical staging really provides only an estimate, and the stage of cancer is overestimated or underestimated in a significant number of cases. More-accurate assessments can be made through pathological staging, which involves directly examining tissues removed in a radical prostatectomy.

C. What Is the Difference between Localized, Locally Advanced, Regionally Advanced, and Advanced or Metastatic Prostate Cancer?

The general names given to various types of cancer are not always agreed on, but as a rule, localized cancer is restricted to the prostate. The terms locally advanced, regionally advanced, and advanced cancer describe cancers that have spread beyond the prostate. Recurring cancer is not one of the stages, and it can be either localized or advanced to some degree.

4

Finding Advanced Prostate Cancer— The Tests from A to Z

Finding Advanced Prostate Cancer—The Tests from A to Z

What Tests Are Used to Find and Understand Prostate Cancer?

There are many ways to diagnose and analyze prostate cancer. However, we must remind you that the only "official" way to diagnose prostate cancer today is through a biopsy.

The following is a list of the currently available tests (and some that seem to be on the verge of becoming available) that are related to prostate cancer. For each, we provide a description, look at any drawbacks, and provide an overall "grade" for the test. In our grading scheme:

▶ A means, yes, you should have this test done if you qualify for it.

▶ B means you should think about having this test done if you qualify for it.

▶ C means no, you should probably not have this test done now. (Some tests in this category may become more useful in the future.)

Alkaline phosphatase

This is a simple blood test. Alkaline phosphatase is an enzyme made in the liver, bones, kidneys, intestines, and placenta. The body produces more of it when the liver and/or bones are being damaged. So, by taking a blood test, doctors can get a sense of the rate of liver and/or bone damage being caused by prostate cancer. This test is usually done for patients who have, or are suspected of having, advanced disease that has spread to the liver and/or bones.

Drawbacks

The liver manufactures a large amount of alkaline phosphatase, so this is not a good early screening test.

Overall grade—B

In cases where cancer has spread to the bone, this test can be useful in measuring the progression of the disease. It is not, however, a good screening test.

Angiogenesis (also called "Microvessel Density or MVD" and "neovascularity")

This test is done on your pathology biopsy. If an area of the body is not getting enough blood, the affected tissue may respond by releasing certain substances that cause blood vessels to grow toward it. That process is called angiogenesis, and it occurs during pregnancy to supply blood to the fetus, or when a wound or tissue is trying to recover from an injury. It can also happen with abnormal tissues. Researchers think that some prostate cancers may rely on angiogenesis to grow, and that by assessing the blood vessels in tissue samples, doctors will be able to tell how far a cancer has spread, and perhaps predict how a cancer may act.

In the angiogenesis test, a pathologist examines tissue removed during surgery, biopsy, or other procedure such as a TURP. The tissue is stained to make blood vessels more visible, and the blood vessels are counted, either manually or by a computer.

If this test turns out to have practical value, it will probably be most useful for cancers that are localized or have spread slightly beyond the prostate. It may also be useful in helping patients who are worried about recurrence after localized cancer treatment.

Probably the most exciting news about angiogenesis is that if researchers can come up with a drug that can inhibit the growth of blood vessels, they may be able to treat the cancer effectively. That means that recently discovered substances, such as angiostatin and endostatin, may turn out to be useful in fighting prostate cancer.

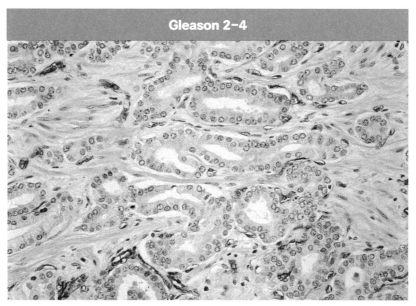

Gleason 2–4

A low grade (Gleason 2-4) or not very aggressive prostate cancer sample stained to see angiogenesis or new blood vessel growth (the dark grey=blood vessels)

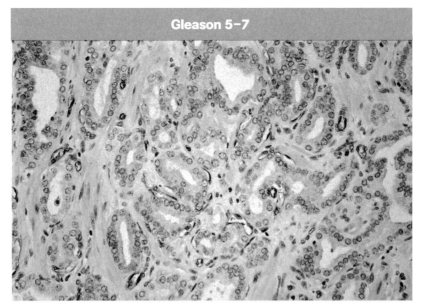

A moderate grade (Gleason 5-7) or moderately aggressive prostate cancer sample stained to see angiogenesis or new blood vessel growth (the dark grey=blood vessels)

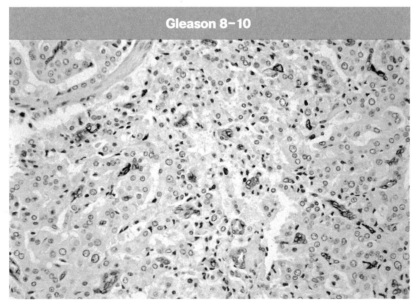

A high grade (Gleason 8-10) or very aggressive prostate cancer sample stained to see angiogenesis or new blood vessel growth (the dark grey=blood vessels)

Drawbacks

More studies are needed to understand whether angiogenesis plays a large role in prostate cancer. Also, we know that some cancers do not need a large blood supply to grow, so angiogenesis tests won't tell us much about those cases. In terms of treatment, most of the drugs that might inhibit angiogenesis have not gone beyond test tube or animal studies.

Overall grade—C

We still have much more to learn about angiogenesis and prostate cancer.

Biopsy of the prostate (also called Transrectal Ultrasound-guided biopsy)

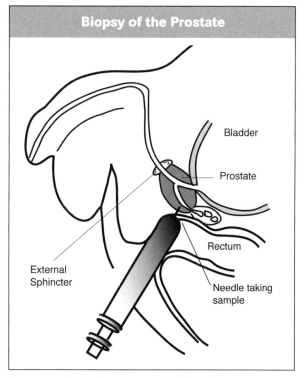

Biopsy of the Prostate

Bladder

Prostate

Rectum

External Sphincter

Needle taking sample

A prostate biopsy is still the best way to determine whether or not cancer exists in the prostate. It can be very helpful in determining whether cancer has spread beyond the prostate. A pathologist can look at the biopsy sample to see if the capsule of the prostate has been penetrated by the cancer, and at tissue from around the prostate to look for signs of locally advanced disease.

In general, a biopsy is appropriate when there is a good possibility of someone having cancer, based on a positive digital rectal exam (DRE), an elevated PSA level and/or a suspicious site on an ultrasound.

A biopsy involves taking a small sample of tissue that is examined by a pathologist to determine whether it is cancerous. An ultrasound probe is inserted in the rectum so that a physician can see the prostate on an ultrasound machine. The probe has a small biopsy needle that can go through the lining of the rectum and into the prostate so that a small piece of tissue (also called a "core") can be removed and examined. While this procedure is uncomfortable, it is brief (a few minutes) and a person can be medicated to relax so the procedure is easier to tolerate.

There are two types of biopsy needles: a 14 gauge needle and a newer, smaller 18 gauge needle. The 18 gauge needle has some advantages, including a reduced chance of post-biopsy infections, a better chance of getting a quality sample, less discomfort, and a decrease in the false negative rate (that is, if no cancer is found there is a good chance that no cancer is actually there). The disadvantage is that it provides less tissue for examination than the 14 gauge needle.

There is some question about how many biopsy samples should be taken at one time. Currently, most doctors take what is called a "sextant" biopsy, which means six pieces of tissue are taken from different areas of the peripheral zone of the prostate. Some doctors may take less and some may take more. For example, some physicians take eight biopsy samples at one time, six from the peripheral zone and two from the transitional zone. And, if the physician suspects that cancer has spread to the seminal vesicles, a biopsy(s) may be taken from there.

We recommend that you ask your physician how many biopsies he or she will take and from what parts of the prostate they will be taken. There is a basic trade-off at work here: The fewer samples taken, the less likely it is that you may experience complications, such as bleeding or infection, from the biopsy—but the chances of missing cancerous tissue increase. The more biopsies taken, the more likely it is that you will experience complications, but you are also more likely to find any cancer that is present.

Drawbacks
The biopsy needle is very tiny compared to the size of the prostate. Therefore, the possibility of missing the cancer does exist. In addition, if cancer is suspected due to a DRE, PSA, or ultrasound, and the biopsy turns up no cancer but does find high-grade PIN, there is a good chance you will have to have the biopsy repeated later on.

Overall grade—A
Again, a biopsy is the only way to officially diagnose prostate cancer. In addition, a biopsy is needed to determine a Gleason score, which tells doctors how aggressive a cancer is.

Bone Scan (also called "radionuclide bone scan" or "radioisotopic bone scan")
A "bone scan" shows whether or not cancer has spread to any of the bones in the body. It is an imaging test that lets doctors take a "picture" of your skeleton. Before the procedure, a harmless dye or isotope—typically something called "Technetium"—

Bone Scan from an Advanced Prostate Cancer Patient

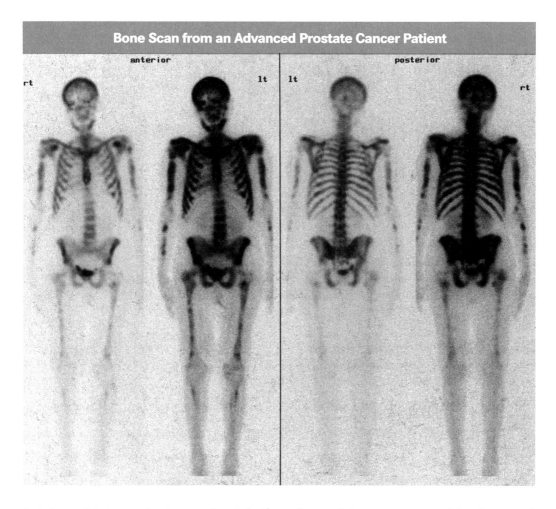

is injected into a vein. Approximately three hours later an x-ray machine is passed around the body and a picture of the bones is taken. This is a painless procedure with the exception of the original needle poke. This dye travels throughout the body and becomes concentrated in areas of the skeleton or bone that may have cancer—areas that are sometimes referred to as "hot spots." However, if a hot spot appears on both sides of the body in the same location, it is usually not an indication of cancer. For example, if there is a spot on the 4th right rib and a spot on the 4th left rib at the same location, then it is probably not cancerous. More likely, it represents arthritis or some other disease. However, if a dark spot appears on the 4th right rib and there is nothing on the left rib, then the hot spot is more likely to indicate the presence of cancer.

This is a good test for anyone suspected of having advanced prostate cancer. You should have it done if you have any or all of the following:

► Bone pain after being diagnosed with prostate cancer.
► Clinical evidence of advanced disease.
► High alkaline phosphatase level (sometimes).
► High Gleason score (8 - 10) at diagnosis.
► PSA greater than 10 at diagnosis.

Once a bone scan test has been performed, it can be used as a basis for comparing and interpreting later bone scans, and identifying changes in the bone over time.

Drawbacks

A bone scan is extremely sensitive, which means it will probably find cancer if it has spread to the bones. However, it may also provide false-positive results, showing that you have cancer when you actually do not. False-positive bone scans can occur among patients with:

► Arthritis
► Bone infections and bone diseases (for example, a disease of the bone called "Paget's disease")
► Inflammatory bone conditions
► Previous bone surgery
► Old bone fractures or healing fractures
► Osteomyelitis
► Trauma to the bones

False-negative results hardly ever occur with a bone scan (less than 1% of the patients tested get such results).

Overall grade: A

This test is invaluable for anyone suspected of having cancer that has spread to the bones. In cases where cancer spread is known, a bone scan provides a tool for seeing whether the bone tumors are decreasing, staying the same, or increasing.

Color Doppler Imaging (also called "CDI" or transrectal color Doppler Imaging)

This is a form of ultrasound testing where an ultrasound probe is placed in the rectum and sound waves are used to produce an image of the prostate. While it is mildly uncomfortable, most men have no problem with the test. Cancer cells need blood, and as they grow, an abnormal flow of blood is often created around the cancer (see "angiogenesis," above). Scientists hope that by being able to detect that flow, they will also be able to detect the cancer it is supplying. That's where Color Doppler Imaging plays a part.

In this test, a special type of transrectal ultrasound probe is inserted into the rectum so that the prostate and the areas around it can be visualized. In the images doctors see, different colors correspond to the degree of blood flow to the cancer. Cancers that have little to no blood flow going to them are given a low number or numbers (such as 0 or +1), and cancers that have a lot of blood flowing to them are given higher numbers (+2 or above).

Color Doppler Imaging is relatively new, but has already been used to find blood vessels feeding breast, kidney, liver, ovary, and rectal cancers. Researchers have recently found that increased blood flow to a prostate cancer can be picked up by this new technique, and may be associated with a higher Gleason score and a higher chance of having cancer in the seminal vesicles. Research also suggests that an increased flow detected with this method may indicate a higher possibility of cancer recurrence after treatment.

Currently, this test is used in prostate patients who are suspected of having locally advanced disease, to help determine treatment options.

Drawbacks

Again, this test is still experimental. We know that it will sometimes show an abnormal blood flow in normal tissue, as well as tissue associated with prostatitis, PIN, and BPH. Also, we are not sure how big a role angiogenesis and blood supply play in all prostate cancers.

Overall grade: C

More research is needed to understand the true value of this test.

CT Scan (usually called a CAT Scan)

This is an x-ray imaging test, in which the person lies on a flat table while a device takes a series of x-rays of the body. The patient is usually injected with a dye to enhance the images, but the test can be done without dye if the person is allergic to it. The procedure itself takes 15 to 45 minutes. Afterward, the x-rays are read by a physician to determine whether anything suggests the presence of cancer. The CT scan is used to look for the presence of cancer in lymph nodes and the liver.

Drawbacks

The CT scan has been a good diagnostic tool in some areas of medicine, but it has been less effective in detecting prostate cancer. Cancers must be fairly large to show up in this test—and cancers that extend beyond the prostate tend to be relatively small, and are often missed. Overall, the CT scans are only 15% - 50% accurate in detecting locally advanced cancer. In assessing lymph nodes, they are accurate 40% - 50% of the time.

Overall grade—A

This test is used routinely in assessing advanced disease.

DNA Ploidy

This test is done using the pathology specimen. It analyzes the DNA from cancer cells obtained in a biopsy or through surgery in order to help determine how aggressive the cancer might be. There are 3 types of DNA that can be found in cells:

▶ Diploid, which is the normal type of DNA .

▶ Aneuploid (also called nondiploid), which is abnormal DNA—there is less or more DNA than normal.

▶ Tetraploid (also called nondiploid), which is abnormal DNA—there is double or twice as much DNA as normal.

There are three techniques used to test DNA ploidy: flow cytometry, static image analysis, and fluorescence in situ hybridization (FISH). These vary in technical detail, but all three strive to provide information that can help stage and grade cancer. For example, some patients with diploid tumors have a greater chance of survival than those with aneuploid or tetraploid tumors.

At this point, DNA ploidy tests are probably most appropriate for people with localized or locally advanced cancer, when doctors want to get some idea of where the disease might go in the future.

Drawbacks

The big problem with this test is that a single prostate tumor can have tissue with different DNA ploidy types. In other words, many patients have tumors with diploid, aneuploid, and tetraploid cells in the same sample, so a test may overestimate or underestimate the aggressiveness of the cancer. In fact, an international ploidy conference recently reviewed all the data on ploidy and determined that it should not be used on a regular basis for prostate cancer at this time.

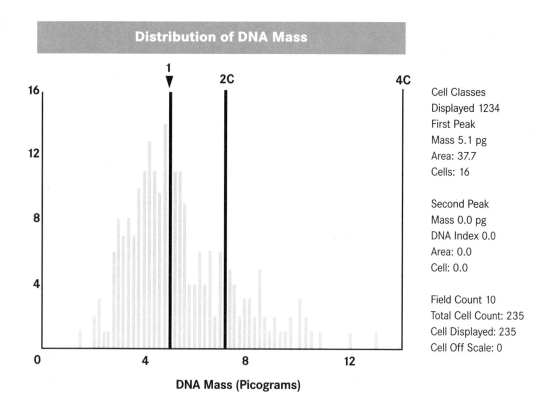

Distribution of DNA Mass

Cell Classes
Displayed 1234
First Peak
Mass 5.1 pg
Area: 37.7
Cells: 16

Second Peak
Mass 0.0 pg
DNA Index 0.0
Area: 0.0
Cell: 0.0

Field Count 10
Total Cell Count: 235
Cell Displayed: 235
Cell Off Scale: 0

DNA Mass (Picograms)

Overall grade—B

Until this test is developed further, it probably doesn't have a lot of value for most patients.

DRE ("Digital Rectal Examination")

In this test, the physician inserts an index finger into the patient's rectum for a few seconds to feel for any hardness, or "induration," on the prostate. If hardness or an abnormality is found, then the test is called a "DRE positive" and the next step is to have a biopsy.

This is still probably the easiest method we have for detecting prostate cancer, and in about 50% of the cases where a DRE indicates the presence of cancer, cancer does indeed show up in a biopsy. A DRE may also be helpful in finding non-cancerous conditions such as BPH or prostatitis.

A DRE should be part of a regular physical examination, along with a PSA test. However, this test can also be useful after someone has been diagnosed with prostate cancer, when the doctor is looking for locally advanced disease. After hormonal treatment, radiation, or cryosurgery, a DRE can help doctors see if the treatment has reduced the size of the tumor in the prostate.

Drawbacks

DREs miss about 20% - 50% of prostate cancers when they are used alone, and more than 50% of the cancers found by DRE alone are actually advanced. That's why a biopsy should be done on all men who have an abnormal DRE.

Another problem is that many physicians disagree on what an abnormal prostate actually feels like, and it is difficult to accurately determine the stage of the cancer through a DRE alone. Therefore, if you are suspected of having locally advanced disease, a DRE alone should never be used to stage your cancer or to tell how far it has spread. In general, a PSA, ultrasound, biopsies, CT scans, and bone scans may be needed to help determine cancer spread. Each patient may be a little different and you should discuss this with your doctor.

Overall grade—A

The DRE is still one of the easiest, cheapest, and most effective ways we have of finding prostate cancer. In addition, it may be able to tell you if your cancer has extended beyond the prostate or if your treatment was successful in reducing the size of your cancer in the prostate.

Free to Total PSA (also called Percent Free PSA or Serum Percent Free PSA)

This is a simple blood test that determines the percentage of Free PSA (fPSA) in your overall PSA. It is generally used when a man has an increase in his PSA, and doctors want to figure out whether cancer or BPH is causing the increase.

A little explanation: PSA is released by the prostate in many different forms, including Free PSA, which is PSA by itself, and ACT PSA, which is PSA attached to a protein. Adding the amount of Free PSA and ACT PSA gives you the Total PSA (Free PSA + ACT PSA=Total PSA).

A few years ago, researchers discovered that men who had a higher percentage of Free PSA were less likely to have cancer than men with a lower percentage of Free PSA. So measuring Free PSA can help determine whether an abnormality in the prostate is cancer or BPH, because men with BPH can be expected to have a higher percentage of Free PSA.

Drawbacks

Currently, this test is used to find localized or confined prostate cancer—it does not tell us much about advanced disease. Recent studies have found no association between Free PSA and grade, stage, or seriousness of disease. In fact, a number of patients with advanced prostate cancer have high percentages of Free PSA, while others have low levels. In addition, an individual's race and/or age may have an effect on his free PSA level.

This is not the end of the story, however. Some studies suggest that the Free PSA percentage significantly increases in patients receiving hormonal or radiation treatments, which may mean that Free PSA could someday be used to gauge the success of such treatments.

Overall grade—B

Although this test is useful in determining the overall presence of cancer, it doesn't provide doctors with any information that can be used to understand advanced prostate cancer.

Hemoglobin Test (Hb Test)

This is a blood test that is commonly done in doctors' offices. Hemoglobin is the molecule that carries oxygen in your blood. If you have a low hemoglobin, you are anemic, and you may become tired or fatigued and short of breath. Doctors working with prostate patients track hemoglobin because some treatments, such as chemotherapy, can lower hemoglobin. Low hemoglobin can be treated with a blood transfusion.

This test is usually done at the start of or during therapy that can lower hemoglobin levels, such as hormone ablation or chemotherapy. Some studies have suggested that a hemoglobin test can be used in predicting who will do well on a certain chemotherapy program, but this has not been proven.

Drawbacks

There are no drawbacks to this test (except that a needle is used to take some blood).

Overall grade—A

This is a routine test that is used regularly.

IGF-1 (Insulin Growth Factor-1)

IGF-1 stands for Insulin Growth Factor-1. Growth factors are released by cells in the body to stimulate cell growth and development. Recent research has shown that men who have higher levels of IGF-1 in their bloodstream may be at an increased risk of being diagnosed with prostate cancer. (It also suggests that women with higher levels of IGF-1 may be at increased risk of getting breast cancer.)

The levels of IGF-1 are assessed through a blood test. In the future, then, men and women may have their IGF-1 level checked to see if they are at increased risk of getting cancer, in much the same way that cholesterol is checked today to gauge a person's risk for heart disease. Currently, this test might be useful if you have a family history of prostate cancer, and the doctor wants more information to help determine your risk of getting the disease.

Drawbacks

This test is not for anyone who has already been diagnosed with prostate cancer, because it simply provides a forward-looking view of risk, rather than useful information about existing disease. Also, there are only a few studies so far that have linked IGF-1 to developing prostate cancer later in life, so much more research needs to be done.

Overall grade—C

This test is still experimental, and really doesn't provide any helpful information in terms of advanced prostate cancer.

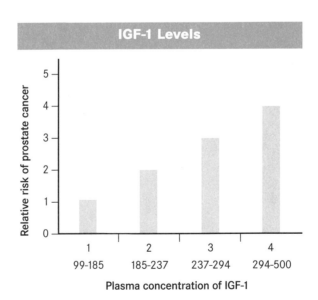

Men with the highest IGF-1 levels have four times the risk of prostate cancer of men with the lower levels.

Laparoscopic Pelvic Lymphadenectomy (also called pelvic lymph node dissection)

When the lymph nodes are invaded by prostate cancer, they often don't become enlarged, making it hard to detect the spread of cancer through CT scans and other tests that look for increased size. As a result, doctors sometimes sample nodes for cancer, removing some tissue in a minor surgical procedure called laparoscopic pelvic lymphadenectomy, or pelvic lymph node dissection (PLND).

There are actually three types of PLND that can be done. These are all types of surgery with varying sizes of incisions. This procedure should be discussed with your urologist. The type of procedure may depend on how many lymph nodes the urologist wants to examine.

- Open pelvic lymph node dissection
- Minilaparotomy for pelvic lymph node dissection (also called "Minilap")
- Laparoscopic pelvic lymph node dissection

In the past, the sampling of the lymph nodes for cancer was only done before radiation or a radical prostatectomy. Today, however, PLNDs are performed as a separate procedure. Typically, this requires a hospital stay of one or two days and the patient can return to work within a week.

This test is mainly for patients who show no evidence of spreading cancer in other tests; who have a long life expectancy; and who have a high Gleason score (8-10) and/or a PSA greater than 20. This test is being used less and less frequently.

Drawbacks

It will still take years to determine how effective this test really is, because it is still fairly new as a separate procedure. Also, this is minor surgery, but it's surgery nonetheless. That means that it takes time and requires a highly skilled urologist, so its use should really be limited to relatively few patients. The Minilap should not be done on obese patients or on men who have had several pelvic surgeries.

Overall grade—B

This may be a good option for some patients; however, it should not be used for every patient.

LDH

This is a simple blood test. LDH stands for "Lactate Dehydrogenase," an enzyme found in the blood and many body organs. An LDH blood test is not a specific test for prostate cancer—it can also be used in monitoring people who are having a heart attack or who have liver disease.

Some studies have suggested that LDH levels go up when a person's prostate cancer is more active. Therefore, some physicians use it to monitor a patient's response to chemotherapy. Others have suggested that LDH, like alkaline phosphatase and hemoglobin, may be useful in predicting the future course of some prostate cancers.

Drawbacks
As a tool for monitoring prostate cancer, LDH tests are unreliable and inconsistent.

Overall grade—C
This test is just not specific enough for prostate cancer.

Monoclonal Antibodies (also called immunoscintigraphy or CYT-356; ProstaScint; or 7E11-C5.3)

This is a painless imaging test that involves the injection of special antibodies with a radioactive imaging agent attached to them into the bloodstream. These antibodies travel through the body and attach themselves to cancer tissues, and the concentrated antibodies show up on an image as dark areas when x-rays or scans are taken of the body.

Two imaging sessions are needed to get results. The first session involves an injection of the antibodies into the bloodstream. About 30 minutes later, a number of pictures (scans) are taken of your body. This procedure usually takes about an hour and provides baseline images for the test.

The patient is then scanned again two to five days later, in order to allow enough time for the previously injected material to concentrate in areas where there may be cancer. The night before this second session, the patient takes an oral laxative, and the next morning receives an enema and empties his bladder—all of which helps in getting a clear picture. Then, scans are taken in a session lasting two or three hours.

Monoclonal antibodies have generated a lot of interest in the past few years. They have been used for some time to find cancers of the colon, ovary, and lungs, and in 1996, a monoclonal antibody called Capromab pendetide (also called CP, and sold under the name ProstaScint) received FDA approval for use in detecting prostate cancer.

Currently, this test is used mainly with patients who:

► have a newly diagnosed prostate cancer that is localized, and who may be at high risk for spread to the lymph nodes, and/or

► have undergone a radical prostatectomy or other curative procedure and are now experiencing a rising PSA with no detectable cancer recurrence through conventional imaging techniques such as CT scans or MRI.

There are several advantages to the monoclonal antibody test.

► It may be effective in confirming that cancer has not spread. It is very specific (it can tell you when cancer is actually not at that location), especially for the detection of lymph node cancer, making it possible to tell patients with a localized disease that it has not spread to the nodes.

► It can detect tumors that are too small to be found by CT scan or MRI.

► It allows doctors to create images of the entire body. The antibodies circulate throughout the body, making them useful in looking for cancer beyond the prostate, in the lymph nodes, or in other organs and tissues.

► The side effects are minimal, occurring in only about 1% - 5% of patients. The most common side effect is temporary increased levels of bilirubin in the blood which are not harmful. Some patients may experience changes in their blood pressure. Most people are able to resume their daily activities immediately after the procedure.

Current research tells us that this test is the most sensitive (it can tell you when cancer is really present) noninvasive tool for detection of lymph node prostate cancer spread (regionally advanced disease), but it is less sensitive than a bone scan in finding cancer that has spread to the bones, and it is probably less sensitive than a CT or MRI in finding cancer that has spread to the liver and spleen.

Drawbacks

The monoclonal antibody test is good, but there are some drawbacks:

► It is not very effective in confirming that you have cancer spread (as opposed to confirming that cancer has not spread, which it is very good at).

► The images are not easy to read. It takes a good deal of experience and some guesswork to determine whether some sites have antibodies attached to them. So, something that looks like cancer may be something else, and vice versa. As doctors become more familiar with the technology, the reading of images may become more precise.

► It uses antibodies from mice. Some individuals (but only a small number)

ProstaScint Scan

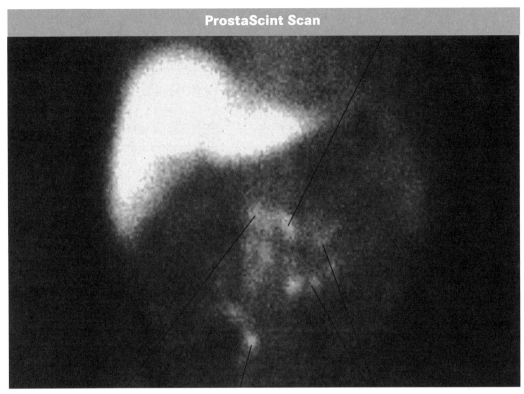

ProstaScint scan that shows lighted areas, which means there may be some cancer in those lymph nodes (the large lighted area at the top of the picture is a normal liver with no cancer. It is lighted up because it usually absorbs a lot of the dye).

are allergic to mouse products. More important, humans develop their own antibodies to these mouse antibodies when the test is used, making follow-up tests less accurate. For example, about 8% of patients develop their own antibodies after the test is used once. If it is used twice, about 19% of the patients develop their own antibodies. So it is important to do this test only in those patients who truly qualify for it.

Overall grade—B
Currently, this is an option for individuals concerned with lymph node spread and/or cancer recurrence after treatment. However, this may change with time—the future is promising for this test.

MRI (magnetic resonance imaging) and endorectal coil MRI

As its name suggests, MRI uses a magnetic field, rather than radiation, to produce images of the body painlessly. During the procedure, a series of images is created while the patient lies in an open tube for 30 to 45 minutes. There is also a new version of this test, called endorectal coil MRI, which uses a small probe inserted into the rectum to take pictures of the prostate and the areas around it.

The MRI offers no advantage over transrectal ultrasound (TRUS) tests in staging more localized cancers. In fact, TRUS has been found to be a better indicator of determining whether cancer has become locally advanced.

The endorectal coil MRI, on the other hand, has produced some interesting results lately. In a recent study, for patients who had a moderately elevated PSA (10-20) and a moderate Gleason score (5-7), the test was able to determine whether the seminal vesicles had cancer more than 95% of the time. However, many more studies are needed to see if this test can provide additional information beyond that which is currently available through PSA, Gleason scores, and other methods.

This test is appropriate for some patients who are believed to have cancer that has spread just beyond the prostate or into the lymph nodes.

Drawbacks

These MRI tests may show cancer where there is none, or fail to show it when it is actually present. Simply put, not enough studies have been completed. Also, these tests are fairly expensive.

Overall grade—B

The good news about these tests is that they are constantly evolving and they seem to be getting better with time.

Neural Networks

This is a computer system that takes a man's clinical information (age, PSA, etc.) and analyzes it in order to determine whether he has cancer, how far it may have spread, and/or what kind of treatment would be best. The system performs this analysis by comparing the patient's data to thousands of previous cases and other medical data.

Drawbacks

Since the information in the computer is based on past data, it may not reflect recent advances in testing or treatment if it is not updated. In addition, we are still not sure which clinical information should be used in the computer analysis.

For example, should race be included? Or, how about newer tests that show promise, but are not yet proven? Medicine is constantly evolving and the computer model has to keep up with changes.

Overall grade—C

This grade is based mostly on the promise of the technology, not the current state of the art. As more and more knowledge is gained about prostate cancer, these computer models may become quite useful.

PAP ("Prostatic Acid Phosphatase")

This blood test, which is not related to the PAP smear used to test for cancer of the cervix, has actually been around for more than 50 years and was widely used before the PSA test was discovered.

The test determines the level of PAP, an enzyme of unknown function, thought to be a marker of prostate cancer, which is released by the prostate and present in the blood.

This test is fairly good at detecting advanced prostate cancer, but not at staging the disease. If the PAP level is elevated, it may point to the spread of cancer beyond the prostate. If the PAP is normal, it doesn't really tell us much, because it could mean that cancer has spread beyond the prostate or is confined to the prostate.

This test is rarely used, having been more or less replaced by the more accurate PSA test. A PAP test may be appropriate before treatment for clinically localized disease (such as surgery) to see if there is any cancer spread beyond the prostate. Also, in some patients suspected of having advanced or metastatic prostate cancer, it may provide doctors with additional insight.

Drawbacks

Some of the problems associated with the PAP test are:

▶ Acid phosphatase is released from other tissues, in addition to the prostate, which can lead to false high readings in the blood test.

▶ The test requires the special handling and processing of a blood sample because acid phosphatase is very unstable. If the test is not done right, the results can be seriously affected.

▶ The amount of PAP released can vary dramatically depending on the time of day, or if the prostate has been handled during a DRE or other procedure—or even randomly. Indeed, there are many situations that can cause an increase in PAP levels:

Prostate Manipulation
Biopsy
Catheterization
DRE
Endoscopy
Surgery
Prostate Diseases
BPH
Infarction
Prostatitis
Urinary Retention
Other Cancers
Cancers that involve liver or bone metastasis
Hairy Cell Leukemia
Hodgkin's Disease
Multiple Myeloma
Polycythemia Vera
Kidney Disease
Chronic glomerulonephritis
Gout
Bone or Skeletal Disease
Osteogenesis Imperfecta
Osteosarcoma
Paget's Disease
Liver Disease
Biliary Tract Obstruction
Cirrhosis
Hepatitis
Other Diseases
Gaucher's Disease
Hyperparathyroidism

Overall grade—C
In the vast majority of cases, a PSA test will be more useful.

Physical Exam
In a physical exam, a physician asks questions about any symptoms that you may have experienced, and examines you to see if you have any pain.

After you have been diagnosed with prostate cancer, you should have any urinary symptoms or pain checked. Indeed, even if you haven't been diagnosed, it's usually a good idea to tell your doctor if you are experiencing any unusual urinary symptoms or physical symptoms, such as swelling in the legs or pelvis, and/or any other pain.

Drawbacks

As we mentioned in an earlier chapter, nearly 90% of the patients with advanced prostate do not have any symptoms. But that also means that 10% do have symptoms.

Overall grade—B

A physical exam can be very helpful in finding any signs of advanced disease.

PSA (Prostate Specific Antigen) Test

This is a simple blood test that measures the amount of PSA in your blood. PSA is a substance produced primarily by the prostate: Essentially, the more PSA released by the prostate, the greater the chance that you might have cancer. In general, 0 - 4 is considered a normal amount, but this can vary. Researchers have tried to cope with such variations by coming up with things such as:

> ▶ Age-Specific Reference Ranges: The normal amount of PSA in the blood as compared to age.
> ▶ PSA Density: The amount of PSA in the blood compared to the size of the prostate by ultrasound measurement.
> ▶ Racial PSA ranges: The normal PSA range among men of different races.
> ▶ PSA velocity: How quickly the PSA increases with time.

This is a good test for men to have as part of their regular checkup. In terms of advanced disease, it is a very useful tool for determining whether treatment has been successful. For example, if you have had your prostate removed, then you should not produce PSA; if you do, there is a good possibility that your cancer has returned. In general, the higher the PSA the greater the chance of having some form of advanced disease. However, PSA alone is not a very good marker for confirming specific clinical staging of a prostate cancer because there are many gray areas in relating PSA values to various cancer stages.

The PSA is also useful in monitoring a response to hormonal or chemotherapy among patients with advanced disease. For example, it is generally accepted that patients who start hormonal therapy should have their PSA level drop to an undetectable level, and patients on chemotherapy should have their PSA decrease.

Drawbacks
PSA can increase due to a number of reasons, including BPH or prostatitis (inflammation or infection of the prostate). In addition, there are some prostate cancers that produce very little PSA (including some very aggressive cancers), so for some individuals a PSA test does not provide a good sense of what is going on.

Overall grade—A
This is the best test that we have for gauging the success of prostate cancer treatment.

Prostate-Specific Membrane Antigen (PSMA)
PSMA is an antigen or protein that is found on the cell surface of prostate cells as well as a few other cell types in the body. An antibody to PSMA is used in the ProstaScint test. It has also been used in RT-PCR reactions.

Drawbacks
It cannot be used as a blood test like PSA. It has not been demonstrated to be a helpful diagnostic or prognostic factor for prostate cancer.

Overall grade—C
The antibody to PSMA is useful but the actual protein is not.

RT-PCR (Reverse Transcriptase-Polymerase Chain Reaction)
This is a usually a blood test, but in a small number of cases it can also be performed using bone marrow and/or lymph node samples. The RT-PCR looks for traces of PSA or prostate-specific membrane antigen (PSMA) in areas of the body that do not normally secrete PSA or PSMA. In other words, it looks for cancer cells that have left the prostate and spread to other parts of the body. This test is still experimental, but in laboratories it has been able to detect the presence of just one prostate cell in a group of 1 million nonprostate cells.

It is important to mention that just because one or several cancer cells have spread beyond the prostate does not necessarily mean that you have advanced disease. The human body is capable of killing cancer cells that have spread.

Drawbacks
This experimental test is still far from perfect. For example, results may vary

from laboratory to laboratory, and some institutions report very good results while others believe the test is not so good—largely because the test is still evolving. It also seems that the test can provide false information: For example, if test results are negative there is a good chance that cancer has not spread, but if it is positive, we cannot be sure that the cancer has actually spread.

Overall grade—C
This test still has a long way to go, but holds some promise.

Seminal Vesicle Biopsy
Locally advanced prostate cancer often involves the seminal vesicles, so some physicians perform biopsies on them. In this test, a small amount of seminal vesicle tissue is removed with a biopsy device (the same type of device used to remove prostate tissue for biopsy).

This test is usually used when doctors suspect that cancer has spread just beyond the prostate. For example, if you have had a treatment such as surgery, radiation, or cryosurgery to treat localized cancer, doctors may want to perform a biopsy on the seminal vesicles to see if cancer is present, and whether further treatments are warranted.

Some physicians believe that seminal vesicle biopsies only detect cancer that has invaded this area to a large degree. Therefore, this test should probably be done primarily among patients who have a PSA greater than 10 or 20.

Drawbacks
The seminal vesicles are small and located near the prostate, so it is difficult for the doctor to know for sure that he or she is accurately taking a tissue sample. Also, cancer may only occupy a small section of the seminal vesicles, so the biopsy may miss it.

Overall grade—B
It is difficult to actually locate the seminal vesicle glands when you try to biopsy them due to their size and location.

Transrectal Ultrasound ("TRUS")
This test uses an ultrasound probe to produce a picture of the prostate and its surroundings. In this case, however, the probe is placed in the rectum, making it possible to get it closer to the prostate. An ultrasound probe is inserted into the rectum so that a physician can see the prostate on an ultrasound machine. While this procedure is uncomfortable, it is brief (a few minutes) and a person can be med-

icated to help relax and tolerate the procedure with ease.

Although there is some discomfort with this test, it has the big advantage of providing a better picture of the prostate and the areas around it. TRUS can not only help doctors diagnose disease, it is also useful in staging prostate cancer and in finding locally advanced disease.

In addition, ultrasound technology is constantly evolving. There is a new addition to the TRUS called "Color Doppler Imaging" (mentioned earlier) or "Tissue Color Flow Mapping." This technique basically allows the physician to get a good idea of the blood flow around the prostate and may help in determining whether a problem is due to cancer or to inflammation (prostatitis).

Drawbacks

TRUS will sometimes indicate that cancer is present when it really isn't, and it may fail to detect cancer when it is actually there. As a rule, this test should be done in conjunction with a DRE and PSA.

Overall grade—B

When used alone, but "A" when used in conjunction with DRE, PSA, and biopsy.

Tumor Associated Gene Tests

These types of tests look at the genes or enzymes associated with the development of cancer. Some genes cause the overgrowth of cells or do not allow cancer cells to die and are activated when a cancer is present. Other genes slow cell growth and are "turned off" when cancer grows. Also, there is an enzyme called telomerase that helps control DNA replication; if it is "turned on," it can keep a cancer growing. To detect such genes and this enzyme, doctors draw a blood sample, stain it, and examine it.

Drawbacks

These tests are still being developed, and have not yet been proven to be reliable and predictable. Doctors hope that they will be useful in differentiating

How p21 - Positive Status Relates to Pathological, Clinical Features of Pca	
Gleason Score	**% Patients p21 - Positive**
2 to 4	57%
5 to 7	53%
8 to 10	65%
pTNM Stage	
T3N0M0 SM-	50%
T3N0M0 SM+	53%
N1 to N2	55%
Bone Metastasis	78%
PSA at Surgery (ng/ml)	
0 to 4	57%
4.1 to 10.0	53%
> 10	69%

Urology Times / Source Alain Maillette, MD

aggressive cancers from more benign ones, and in predicting whether cancer will recur.

Overall grade—C

These tests may become highly valuable as they are improved.

TURP Biopsy

A TURP biopsy is taken during a procedure known as Transurethral Resection of the Prostate, or TURP. A TURP is used to treat serious cases of BPH, or enlarged prostate. During the procedure, patients receive a general or spinal anesthesia, and the physician inserts a long, thin instrument (a resectoscope) into the urethra and on into the bladder. The physician can look through this instrument to get a clear view and use it to cut away excess prostate tissue. The tissue fragments fall into the bladder and a stream of fluid flushes through the resectoscope and out of the body. A sample of this prostate tissue is then sent to the laboratory to be checked for evidence of prostate cancer.

Drawbacks

There are not that many opportunities to gather samples via TURP, because patients can often be treated for BPH by supplements, medication, or other procedures. Also, many patients who have prostate cancer do not have severe BPH that requires a TURP.

Overall grade—B

A TURP is not a diagnostic procedure for cancer; however, during the course of a TURP, cancerous tissue may be found.

X-ray

X-rays are simple—and for most people, familiar—tests. X-rays play a fairly small role in diagnosing prostate cancer, being used primarily to determine whether a person's disease has spread to other parts of the body.

Drawbacks

For the most part, this test is only useful if the physician suspects cancer has spread to the lungs—a situation that occurs in a small number of patients.

Overall grade—B

If you qualify for this test, it can be useful.

5

When Treatment for Localized Cancer Fails (Recurrence)

In this chapter:

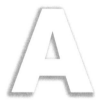

How Do Doctors Evaluate the Effectiveness of Various Treatments?

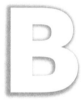

Why Didn't My Treatment for Localized Cancer Work?

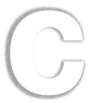

What Are My Treatment Options When Cancer Recurs?

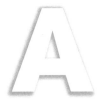

How Do Doctors Evaluate The Effectiveness of Various Treatments?

Doctors have several ways of gauging how successful a particular prostate cancer treatment is. These are often called "end points" because they describe the end outcome of treatment. These end points usually look at treatment in one of two ways:

► 1. The percentage of men receiving the procedure who can expect a successful outcome.
► 2. The percentage of men receiving the procedure who can expect an outcome that is not successful.

If you are thinking about having a procedure done, you should ask the doctor who will perform it and ask about his or her specific end points—that is, how successful they have been with the procedure. Then, you can compare those end points with the average end points from the medical literature.

However, there are a couple of important things to bear in mind. For one, many of the procedures used to treat prostate cancer are fairly new, so they may not have established much of a long-term record. Also, procedures are evolving all the time, so past results may not provide a completely accurate view of the future.

Above all, remember that these end points are statistics that tend to describe the "average" person. These statistics are often based on a wide variety of cases and on predictions and probabilities, and they rely on studies that cover varying lengths of time. Statistics can be helpful in making decisions about treatment, but remember: They can never predict precisely what will happen to you.

There are many end points used by doctors today. Some of the more common ones are as follows:

► Overall survival rates.

Basically, this indicates how long individuals usually live after a given treatment, and it includes any cause of death. For example, if a person lives for 20 years after prostate cancer surgery and dies of heart disease or is hit by a car, he is counted. Therefore, this is not a very precise assessment of the success of a procedure.

► Cancer-specific survival rates (also called cancer survival).

This looks at the people who die of cancer after being treated for it. For example, if the cancer-specific survival rate for a procedure is 50% at 10 years, it means that the average man who receives this procedure can expect to survive at least 10 years before he dies from prostate cancer. This is a more precise way to describe the effectiveness of a procedure than the overall survival rate.

► Freedom from metastasis, or metastatic-free disease.

This end point looks at how long the average man can expect to be free from advanced disease after a procedure. For example, if 95% of the men receiving this procedure have freedom from metastasis for 15 years, this indicates that it's very effective. It also means that 5% of the men who have this procedure can expect to experience metastasis within 15 years.

► Freedom from local recurrence.

This looks at the length of time after a procedure that someone can expect to be free of localized cancer. For example, you might hear that 80% of the individuals studied had freedom from local recurrence after 10 years, which is pretty good. The use of this measurement suggests that the procedure was performed with the hope of eliminating all of the cancer.

► Freedom from any recurrence.

This is the percentage of individuals who did not have a recurrence of cancer after a certain period of time, or the length of time after a procedure that it typically takes for signs of recurring cancer to appear.

► Freedom from biochemical or PSA recurrence (also called biochemical relapse-free survival, detectable PSA, or subclinical progression).

The PSA level should be zero after surgery or close to zero after a procedure such as radiation, so this end point assesses how long it takes for PSA levels to become detectable again (the rise of PSA levels suggests that the cancer has returned). This is probably the most accurate way to gauge the success of prostate cancer treatments, since a rising PSA will often show up long before other clinical signs, such as a positive DRE, bone scan, or serum acid phosphatase levels—as long as three to six years before, in some cases.

It is important to note that the meaning of "freedom from PSA recurrence" can vary depending on the individual doctor or the procedure in question. For example, after a radical prostatectomy you should expect an undetectable PSA or one that is nearly zero (some say less than or equal to 0.2). After a radiation procedure, or other treatment, on the other hand, the PSA level used to determine freedom from PSA recurrence varies from doctor to doctor.

▶ Progression-free survival.

This looks at the percentage of people who can expect to have their cancer remain at the same stage—that is, not advance any further—after a procedure.

▶ Partial and complete disease regression.

Regression literally means "going back," so this is the percentage of individuals who can expect to have their cancer regress somewhat or completely after the procedure or treatment. It is generally used in regard to treatment with hormones or chemotherapy. Reports might show that five years after treatment, 75% of the men with cancer in the nodes had partial or complete disappearance of that cancer—which is a pretty good record. It is important to keep in mind that there is a difference between partial and complete regression. Partial regression means that the cancer is still in a certain location in the body, but there is less of it than there was prior to the procedure. Complete regression means that the cancer is no longer at that site after the procedure.

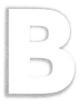

Why Didn't My Treatment for Localized Cancer Work?

There are a number of treatments for localized cancer, including "watchful waiting," surgery, and various types of radiation. These treatments can fail for a variety of reasons. Sometimes the cancer has already spread beyond the area of treatment and this cannot be seen on any tests. However, any treatment is more likely to fail if a person's situation involves any of the following:

▶ Capsular penetration
▶ High-grade cancer (Gleason score of 8 or higher)
▶ Seminal vesicle invasion
▶ Positive margins

There is some debate about the last point because some studies show that positive margins are not important in determining whether cancer will recur, while other studies suggest that they do. To be on the safe side, we've included the "positive margins" item in our list. Also, remember that these four factors do not mean for certain that cancer will recur. Some treatments will fail without any of the above conditions being present, and some patients with all of them will have successful treatment.

The table below shows the percentage of men with certain conditions that are likely to have a detectable PSA after five years.

Condition	Detectable PSA at five years
Capsular penetration	5-35% of men
Positive margins	50-70% of men
Seminal vesicle invasion	35-65% of men
High-grade (Gleason 8,9, or 10) cancer	55-95% of men

Why didn't watchful waiting work?

Watchful waiting is just that—watching and waiting. This approach has many names, such as:

▶ Conservative therapy
▶ Delayed therapy
▶ Expectant management
▶ No therapy
▶ Surveillance
▶ Without specific therapy

Why does watchful waiting sometimes fail? Simple—you are not doing anything to the cancer other than monitoring it with tests such as PSA. Therefore, you are allowing the tumor to grow. This approach is sometimes taken because many patients with low-stage cancers have tumors that will grow very slowly. In some cases, these tumors may never show symptoms. In addition, many patients with prostate cancer are older and have other more serious diseases to worry about.

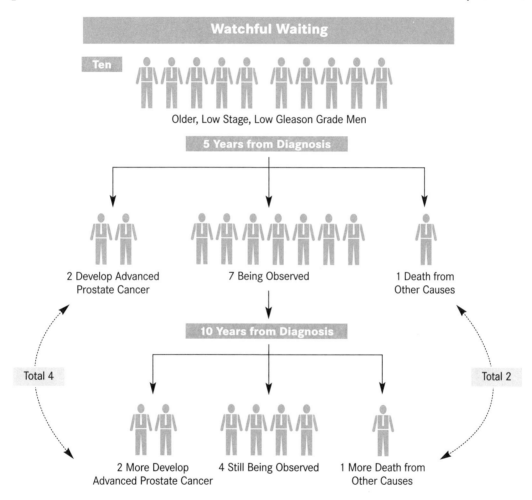

Watchful Waiting

Ten

Older, Low Stage, Low Gleason Grade Men

5 Years from Diagnosis

2 Develop Advanced Prostate Cancer

7 Being Observed

1 Death from Other Causes

Total 4

10 Years from Diagnosis

Total 2

2 More Develop Advanced Prostate Cancer

4 Still Being Observed

1 More Death from Other Causes

We have a good idea of how well watchful waiting works, in terms of "cancer-specific survival":

▶ Among men with a low total Gleason score (2-4), 2% die of cancer within five years, and 10% within 10 years.

► Among men with a moderate total Gleason score (5-7), 3% die of cancer after five years, and 13% after 10 years.

► Among men with high total Gleason score (8-10), 33% die of cancer after 5 years and 66% will die after 10 years.

Basically, the lower your Gleason score, the more likely it is that watchful waiting will succeed.

In terms of "metastasis-free survival" and watchful waiting, we see the following results:

► Among men with low-grade cancer, only 7% have metastasis after five years, and 19% within 10 years.

► Among men with moderate-grade cancer, 16% have metastasis within five years, and 42% within 10 years.

► Among men with high-grade cancer, 49% have metastasis after five years, and 74% with 10 years.

Why didn't surgery work?

Like Watchful Waiting, surgery also has several names, including radical prostatectomy (the most common name), radical perineal prostatectomy, radical retropubic prostatectomy, and surgical therapy.

The goal of surgery is to remove all of the cancer. It may not work because:

► The cancer has already spread to other locations before the operation. Although doctors can give you a good idea of where your cancer is located, they cannot be 100% accurate. The disease may have spread beyond the prostate—and therefore beyond the reach of the surgical procedure—without the surgeon's knowledge.

► The localized cancer was not completely removed or "excised." During surgery, the surgeon removes the prostate and some surrounding tissue in order to make sure all the cancer is eliminated. However, it is possible that some of the cancer may have grown beyond the areas that the surgeon removes. As mentioned earlier, doctors look for positive surgical margins in removed tissue to check for cancer that extends beyond the area taken out during surgery.

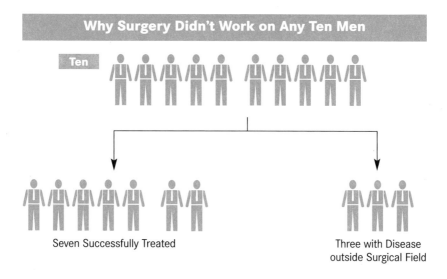

Why Surgery Didn't Work on Any Ten Men

Ten

Seven Successfully Treated

Three with Disease
outside Surgical Field

The special case of a rising PSA after a radical prostatectomy:
Unfortunately, radical prostatectomy is not always successful in curing cancer.
This may be due to microscopic disease that was not removed at the time of surgery. The cancer then begins once more to grow as a local recurrence. If there is no evidence of distant metastases (negative bone scan, negative CT scan), radiation should be considered as a curative salvage treatment. Studies have demonstrated that radiation works better the lower the PSA (<1 - 2).

Why didn't radiation work?

There are basically two types of radiation treatment. The first type is delivered from outside the body or from an external source, and includes:

> ► 3-dimensional (3D) conformal beam radiation
> ► external beam radiation
> ► external beam radiotherapy
> ► neutron beam radiation
> ► proton beam radiation
> ► radical radiation

The second type of radiation can be delivered from inside the body from an internal source. This can be called:

► brachytherapy
► interstitial radiotherapy
► interstitial seed implants
► permanent seed implants
► radioactive seed implants
► seed implants
► temporary seed implants

With both types of radiation, the goal is to kill all the cancer cells without harming normal cells. External beam radiation is the standard first line therapy for treatment of known locally advanced prostate cancer at the time of diagnosis. The most common type of radiation is external beam. It is delivered in the same way as for patients with localized prostate cancer. Patients receive approximately 35 treatments over the course of 7 weeks, with weekends off. For this treatment, patients are placed on a table and the radiation beams are pointed at the area of treatment. Each session only takes 15 to 20 minutes and is painless. Side effects to radiation may include impotence, incontinence, urination frequency, fatigue, and painless rectal bleeding. In general, radiation is well tolerated.

However, radiation can fail for a couple of reasons:
► Not all of the cancer cells were killed, either because they were not hit by the radiation beam or they continued to live even after they were hit by the beam.
► Some of the cancer cells spread beyond the prostate before the procedure was done.
► Other cells in the prostate became cancerous after the procedure was completed.

Survival rates for radiation vary depending on the type of cancer, but overall they are similar to those of radical prostatectomy. In general, about 30% - 40% of the patients receiving radiation will experience an increase in their PSA levels within five years of having the procedure. This also means that the majority will not experience a PSA increase within five years.

If we look at seed implants alone, the vast majority of patients do not experience an increase in their PSA for at least five to seven years after their procedure.

Both procedures have undergone a significant change in recent years, and are now much more accurate and reliable; therefore, these statistics should change for the better as time goes on. In addition, there is new data indicating that men who receive hormonal ablation during and after radiation may stay disease-free for a longer time. So, ask your doctor about hormonal ablation in conjunction with radiation.

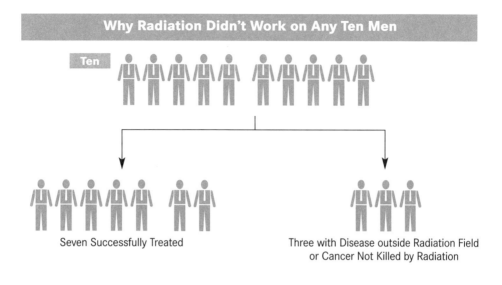

Why Radiation Didn't Work on Any Ten Men

Ten

Seven Successfully Treated

Three with Disease outside Radiation Field or Cancer Not Killed by Radiation

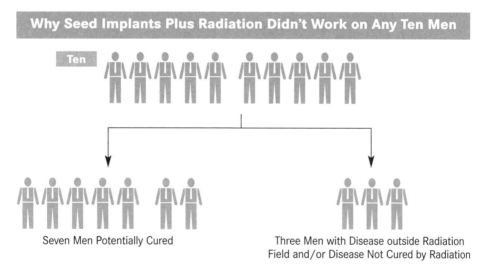

Why Seed Implants Plus Radiation Didn't Work on Any Ten Men

Ten

Seven Men Potentially Cured

Three Men with Disease outside Radiation Field and/or Disease Not Cured by Radiation

Notes on neutron and proton radiation

Like an x-ray, standard radiation uses high-energy photons that pass through the body, imparting energy to anything in the way of the beam. The power in the beam itself decreases as it goes through the body, leaving most of its energy in the first tissues or area it hits. As a result, standard radiation is most useful for cancers near the surface of the body. The deeper inside the body the cancer is (like prostate

Photons
(No Charge and Mass)

Neutrons
(Negative Charge with Mass)

Protons
(Positive Charge with Mass)

cancer), the stronger the beam needed to get to it, and the larger the dose of radiation the healthy tissue absorbs—which increases unwanted side effects.

Neutron and proton radiation are relatively new treatments, but they have been approved by the FDA and are covered by Medicare and most other health insurance companies.

Like standard radiation, these therapies are most effective for cancers lying close to the body surface. Neutron and proton therapies use particles (neutrons and protons, of course) that have different qualities than the photons used in standard therapy. For example, they only go a limited distance into the body, rather than passing through, and that distance can be determined by the starting energy of the particle. The greater the starting energy, the farther into the body it goes. Also, the amount of energy neutrons and protons deliver increases as they slow down, and they give off a large burst of energy when they stop. So unlike standard radiation therapy, where the maximum dose is found at the surface, in neutron and proton treatment, the maximum dose can be placed inside the cancer itself, decreasing the damage to the healthy tissue of the body. This allows the use of far greater doses of radiation to be delivered to the cancer without an increase in side effects.

Neutron radiation

Today, there are only a few places in the U.S. that perform neutron therapy, but as time goes on, more institutions may offer it as an option.

The usual treatment with neutron radiation takes one to two months, with treatments given Monday through Friday for 15 - 30 minutes each time. Treatment is similar to regular external beam radiation where a patient lies on a table and radiation beams are aimed at the patient. These treatments are painless.

Neutron and Neutron/Photon radiation does have side effects, and they increase with the dosage of radiation. Typical side effects may include difficulties with urination such as frequency, urgency, and incontinence. Hip stiffness may develop as late as five years after treatment (data provided by Dr. Jeffrey Foreman at the Barbara Ann Karmanos Cancer Center-Wayne State University). The following photographs is the machine used for neutron treatment.

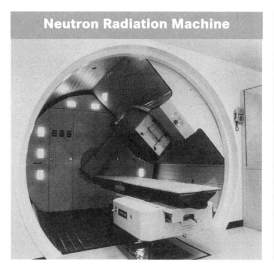

Neutron Radiation Machine

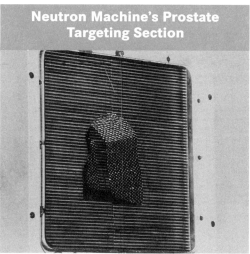

Neutron Machine's Prostate Targeting Section

Proton radiation

Proton radiation's ability to specifically target a dose to the cancer has been useful for treating eye, brain, and spine cancers, where damage to the surrounding area can be very dangerous. However, there have not been many clinical trials of this treatment that involve other areas of the body.

Currently, Massachusetts General Hospital in Boston and Loma Linda University Medical Center in Loma Linda, California, are working together on clinical trials of proton radiation and prostate cancer.

Why didn't cryosurgery work?

Cryosurgery involves the insertion of probes into the prostate through the perineum and killing cancer cells by freezing them. These probes freeze the prostate with the help of ultrasound guidance. This procedure can be uncomfortable, but the patient is given anesthesia so that it is well tolerated. It fails because of a combination of why surgery and radiation fail. First, the cancer cells may have already escaped the area being frozen, and second, the actual freezing may not be enough to kill the cancer cells

The results from cryosurgery seem to be similar to the results of surgery, and the technique has been improving over the last few years; however, there are no long-term data about its effectiveness. However, about a quarter of the patients who receive cryosurgery will experience an increase in their PSA within three to five years after treatment.

A Complete Description of Proton Therapy for Prostate Cancer

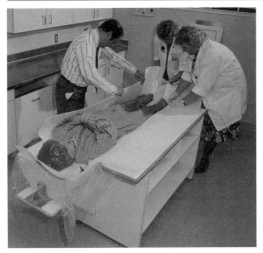

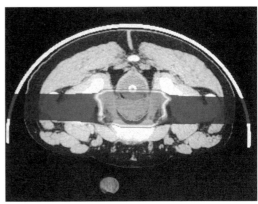

To prepare for accurate proton therapy, a whole body mold is made.

The patient has a CT scan done to identify the prostate target. Note the water-filled balloon inserted into the rectum. This pushes the rectal wall away from the treatment area. The prostate and surrounding normal structures are outlined on each CT scan picture.

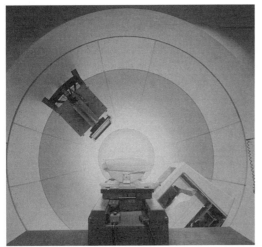

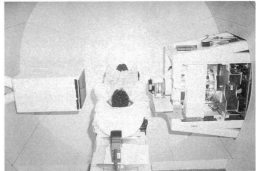

This is a view inside the treatment room. The beam can be delivered from a number of different angles to ensure accurate targeting of the prostate.

This shows the patient in position before treatment begins. For prostate cancer the patient will have 30–40 sesions, which is similar to the number given during standard (photon) radiation.

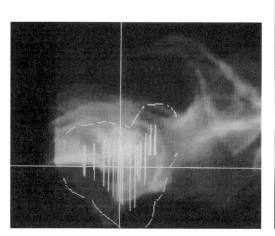
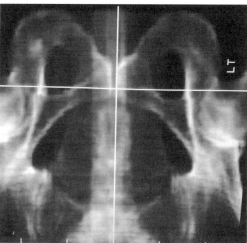

Before each treatment the patient is lined up for targeting with digitally reconstructed x-rays developed from the prior (before the first treatment) CT scan. The patient is moved into the exact position before each treatment, using bone measurements and other internal markers. This helps to hit less normal tissue and more cancerous tissue.

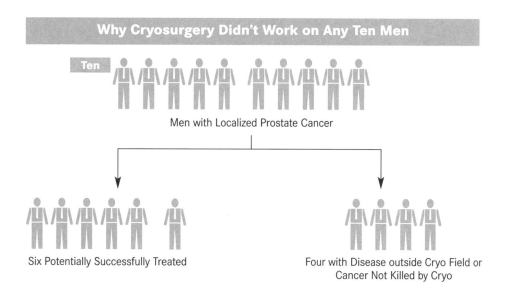

Why Cryosurgery Didn't Work on Any Ten Men

Ten

Men with Localized Prostate Cancer

Six Potentially Successfully Treated

Four with Disease outside Cryo Field or Cancer Not Killed by Cryo

Why didn't hormonal ablation work?

Hormonal ablation is essentially the elimination of hormones. This can be done in a number of ways:

> ► the testicles can be removed
> ► an LHRH injection can be given
> ► an antiandrogen pill can be given
> ► an antiandrogen pill can be given after the testicles have been removed
> ► an LHRH injection can be given along with an antiandrogen pill (or the pill can come later).

LHRH injections can be given every month, every three months, or every four months depending on what the doctor and patient are most comfortable with. There are two types of injections: The Lupron injection, which is usually given in the buttocks or hip, and the Zoladex injection which is usually injected in the abdomen. These injections only take seconds to deliver the LHRH medicine, and they both work about the same.

Hormonal ablation is sometimes used by itself for patients who have undergone watchful waiting; however, it is more often used before, during, or after another treatment, such as radiation.

Common Names for Hormonal Ablation

Hormonal ablation can be performed in a variety of ways, so you may hear it described by a variety of names:

> ► Adjuvant Hormonal therapy or treatment (given after another procedure)
> ► Adjuvant and Neoadjuvant therapy or treatment (given before, during, and after a procedure)
> ► Androgen ablation
> ► Androgen blockade
> ► Androgen deprivation
> ► Antiandrogen treatment
> ► Bilateral orchiectomy (also known as medical castration)
> ► Combined Hormonal Treatment
> ► Double agent androgen deprivation
> ► Hormonal therapy and hormonal treatment (These terms are commonly used, but are somewhat inaccurate, because doctors are not providing hormones, they are eliminating them.
> ► LHRH treatment

- Maximal Androgen Blockade (MAB)
- Monotherapy
- Neoadjuvant Hormonal therapy or treatment (given before a certain procedure)
- Single agent androgen deprivation

Hormonal ablation aims to kill cancer cells that depend on male hormones. The only problem with this method is that some cancer cells do not need hormones to survive, and so are not affected by hormonal ablation (as mentioned in Chapter 2). Thus, this treatment can fail if the cancer in question involves such cells, because any cancer cell that does not depend on hormones will not be killed.

A tumor becomes insensitive to hormonal ablation. Every tumor contains some hormone-sensitive (androgen dependent=AD) cells and some hormone-insensitive (androgen independent=AI) cells. After hormonal ablation, the AD cells die (and the PSA decreases), but the AI cells continue to grow. Eventually, the tumor contains only AI cells; it continues to grow, and the PSA continues to rise despite the hormone ablation. At this point, the cancer is said to be "hormone refractory," or no longer able to respond to the removal of hormones.

Hormonal Ablation in Ten Men

Ten

2 years

Five men experiencing androgen
deprivaton failure ADF

Five men continue in remission for
another year (3 years total)

Two more men experiencing
ADF

Three men continue in remission
for another year (4 years total)

One more man experiencing
ADF

Two men continue in remission for
another year (5 years total)

1 more man
(9 / 10 total)
experiencing ADF

1 man continues
in remission for
indefinite period

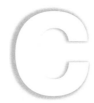

What Are My Treatment Options after Recurrence?

There are many possible therapies that have been approved and/or are experimental for all of the different stages of prostate cancer. Below is a summary of all of the possible treatment options at any stage of cancer or when recurrence occurs.

Standard	Localized	Recurrence	Locally Advanced	Regionally Advanced	Advanced (androgen dependent)	Advanced (androgen independent)
Chemo Rx						✔
External Beam XRT	✔	✔	✔			
Hormonal Rx		✔	✔	✔	✔	
Local XRT						✔
Proton Radiation	✔	✔	✔			
Palliative Care						✔
Radical Prostatectomy	✔		✔			
Strontium 89						✔
Watchful Waiting	✔	✔	✔	✔	✔	
Experimental	Localized	Recurrence	Locally Advanced	Regionally Advanced	Advanced (androgen dependent)	Advanced (androgen independent)
Antibody Therapy						✔
Chemo +XRT	✔					

Experimental (continued)	Localized	Recurrence	Locally Advanced	Regionally Advanced	Advanced (androgen dependent)	Advanced (androgen independent)
Chemo + RRP	✔					
Cryo	✔	✔				
Dietary	✔	✔	✔	✔	✔	✔
Supplement Tx	✔	✔	✔	✔	✔	✔
External Beam	✔	✔	✔	✔		
XRT + Implant	✔	✔	✔	✔		
Gene Therapy						✔
Hormonal Rx	✔					
Hormonal Rx + Exp. Chemo					✔	
Implant XRT	✔		✔			
Immunotherapy						✔
Investigational Chemotherapy						✔
Neutron Radiation	✔		✔			
Proton Radiation			✔			
Radical Prostatectomy			✔			
Vaccine	✔	✔	✔	✔	✔	✔

Please note: Several of the treatment options listed in the above chart are discussed in later chapters of this book. Please refer to the index for page numbers.

6

Diagnosis and Treatment of Advanced Prostate Cancer

In this chapter:

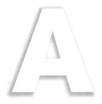

How Can Doctors Find and Treat Locally Advanced Cancer (T3 and T4 Disease)?

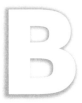

How Can Doctors Find and Treat Regionally Advanced Prostate Cancer (N1 Disease)?

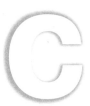

How Can Doctors Find and Treat Advanced Prostate Cancer (D2 or M1 Disease)?

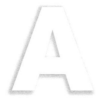

How Can Doctors Find and Treat Locally Advanced Cancer (T3 and T4 Disease)

As we discussed earlier, cancer that has spread just beyond the prostate—to an area near, but outside, the prostate—is known as T3 or T4, or Stage C, prostate cancer. In discussions of such locally advanced disease, you may hear a number of terms, such as capsular penetration or perforation, nonmetastatic prostate cancer, and periprostatic cancer.

Under the newer staging system, there are two types of T3 cancer:
▶ T3a. Cancers that have grown beyond the prostate on one side only (also called "unilateral extracapsular extension").
▶ T3b. Cancers that have grown beyond the prostate on both sides (also called "bilateral extracapsular extension").

T4 cancer has spread to structures near the prostate (other than the seminal vesicles) such as the bladder neck, external sphincter, levator muscles, pelvic wall, and/or rectum.

Some of the names given to T3 or T4 (stage C) stage prostate cancer are:

▶ Capsular penetration
▶ Capsular perforation
▶ Extracapsular penetration
▶ Extracapsular extension (also called "ECE"; it means that cancer has spread just beyond the prostate capsule)
▶ Locally advanced disease

- Locally more than T2 cancer.
- Nonmetastatic prostate cancer
- Periprostatic cancer or disease (indicates that the cancer has grown beyond the prostate and has invaded the tissue right next to it)
- Recurrent prostate cancer
- Seminal Vesicle Invasion (SVI)
- Seminal Vesicle Involvement
- $T3N_0M_0$
- $T4N_0M_0$

Locally advanced cancer can present in two ways. First, it can be present at the initial diagnosis. Second, locally advanced cancer can present as a recurrence because it was not cured by the initial therapy or it may simply have been missed in earlier tests. In fact, some studies report that 20% - 50% of the patients who received localized treatment that failed may have actually had locally advanced disease at the time of diagnosis. Recurrent cancer usually presents itself as a rising PSA.

Diagnosing locally advanced cancer

Most patients with T3 disease have one or more of the following:

> a biopsy that reveals a moderately differentiated (Gleason score of 5,6, or 7) to poorly differentiated (Gleason score of 8,9, or 10) cancer.
> a DRE that suggests that the cancer has extended beyond the prostate.
> a much higher than normal PSA (greater than 20).
> a transrectal ultrasound that suggests that cancer has extended beyond the prostate, along with a negative pelvic CT scan, a negative ProstaScint scan, and a negative bone scan—results that indicate that the cancer has not spread far beyond the prostate.

Of the tests described in Chapter 4, the following are most likely to be useful in diagnosing locally advanced disease:

Biopsy

A biopsy of the prostate is part of the diagnostic workup for prostate cancer. If you have had surgery to remove your prostate as initial treatment, a biopsy may or may not play a role in deciding whether you have had a local recurrence. This is most often decided by the urologist and radiation oncologist.

► Bone Scan

This is done to rule out metastases in your bones and is performed at initial diagnosis or at the time of recurrence.

► CT Scan

This is done to look at the area around your prostate, your lymph nodes, and your liver. Some doctors only get a pelvic CT which looks at the lymph nodes and prostate area and others get an abdominal CT too, which looks at the liver area. This is up to the physician, based on your individual case. It is done at the time of diagnosis if you have a high PSA or high Gleason score. It is also done at the time of recurrence to look for metastatic spread.

► DRE

The digital rectal exam is part of your life once you have prostate cancer. Doctors use it for diagnosis as well as to look for recurrence.

► Monoclonal Antibody Imaging

The ProstaScint scan is generally not done as part of the staging workup at initial diagnosis. It can be useful in determining if recurrent cancer has spread beyond the local prostate bed.

► PSA

Just like the DRE, a PSA is now a part of your life. At diagnosis, a higher PSA is more suggestive of advanced disease. After therapy, PSA is used to monitor for recurrence as well as to monitor the results of therapy.

► Seminal Vesicle Biopsy

This is occasionally done to determine if prostate cancer has spread to the seminal vesicles. It is not a common test.

► Transrectal Ultrasound

The TRUS is part of the diagnostic workup for prostate cancer and is generally done to look for a prostate cancer nodule and to guide the prostate biopsies.

Treatments for Locally Advanced Cancer

Watchful waiting

Watchful waiting is used in relatively few patients with locally advanced cancer. However, it can be an option for older patients with a life expectancy of less than 10 years and low to moderate Gleason scores.

The data on watchful waiting and locally advanced cancer are fairly limited for these types of patients, but research on these men (primarily between the ages of 65 - 80) suggests the following:

Percentage Not Dying of Prostate Cancer		
5 Years	10 Years	15 Years
90-100%	60-90%	50-60%

Progression-Free Survival (% where cancer does not advance)		
5 Years	10 Years	15 Years
20-30%	30-40%	40-50%

In some watchful-waiting studies of patients with stage C or T3/T4 disease, the risk of developing distant metastatic disease for patients with low or moderate Gleason cancers has actually been equal to that of patients receiving initial local therapy. Patients with high-grade cancers are more likely to benefit from treatment. The decision to undergo watchful waiting must be undertaken very carefully, taking into account the wishes of the patient, the age of the patient, and the Gleason score of the tumor. It is an individual decision for each patient and it is difficult to describe the "average" watchful waiting patient.

Radiation

Over the past two decades, radiation therapy has been the most common treatment for locally advanced cancer. Years ago, such treatment was thought to be quite effective, and able to control prostate cancer in 50% to 70% of patients. However, with more accurate testing methods such as PSA at our disposal, we now think it is less effective. The biochemical disease-free survival progression of standard radiation patients after 10 years, for example, is only in the neighborhood of 20% (biochemical disease-free survival rate means that the PSA never goes up). Radiation, however, may provide control of the cancer for the rest of a patient's life. Doctors, however, have developed a couple of methods that can increase the effectiveness of traditional radiation treatments: Dose escalation and hormonal ablation.

Dose escalation

With dose escalation, the dose of radiation is increased to the point where the chances of eliminating cancer are also increased. This sounds simple enough, but in practice it can get complicated, because a dose that is too high can result in severe side effects. That means that doctors have to use special techniques (usually referred to as 3-dimensional conformal planning) to more accurately target the radiation, and avoid damaging healthy tissues near the cancer.

There has not been a lot of research done on dose escalation and locally advanced cancer. However, in one study that we know of, patients with T3 cancer did seem to do better with higher doses. Although this one study cannot be regarded as conclusive proof, it does provide some insight into the possible benefit of increasing radiation dosages. Also, as targeting improves over time, the possibility of successful treatment with minimal side effects is a growing possibility.

Hormonal ablation and radiation

When hormonal ablation (described in Chapter 5) is used in conjunction with radiation, it may increase the effectiveness of treatment. It can be given in the neoadjuvant setting (prior to the start of radiation), the concurrent setting (during radiation), and the adjuvant setting (after radiation). Why would these help? There are a number of possibilities:

> It may reduce the number of cancer cells that have to be eliminated by radiation.
> Apoptosis, or cell death, may be enhanced.
> It may cause cancer cells to be more dependent on oxygen, and also make these cancer cells more likely to be killed by radiation (photon radiation is better at killing cancer cells that depend on oxygen).
> It may cause cancer cells to stop dividing and to stop reproducing so that the cancer is more likely to be killed by radiation.

Neoadjuvant and concurrent: A study done in the 1970s using DES (an estrogen) prior to radiation therapy for locally advanced cancers showed an almost 20% higher rate of local control, compared to radiation therapy alone. Other studies using other hormones (LHRH agonist and an antiandrogen) before and during radiation therapy found 25% better control rates for cancer than radiation therapy alone.

However, the best length of time to use hormonal therapy in conjunction with radiation is not yet known. Some studies are now extending neoadjuvant therapy from three months to eight months before therapy, and the early findings seem to suggest improved results for patients undergoing the longer therapy. Most of these studies keep the patient on hormone ablation while the radiation is given.

Concurrent and adjuvant therapy: In 1998, a study showed that men with T3 and T4 prostate cancer may keep cancer away longer and live longer if they are given hormonal ablation as soon as radiation is started, and then for three years after treatment. In this study:

► about 80% of the men receiving combined treatment were alive five years after treatment, versus a little more than 60% of the men receiving only radiation.

► of the patients who were alive after five years, 85% had no signs of disease, versus 48% of those who only received radiation.

This appears to be great news for men with locally advanced prostate cancer, but more research is needed if we are to know for sure. Also, there are some things to remember when considering those results. For example:

► The men in the study were either given radiation or radiation with hormonal ablation. There were no patients in the study who received hormonal ablation alone. It could be that patients will do just as well on hormonal ablation with no other treatment.

► The study only followed patients for about four years—the rest of the data was based on estimates.

► Men who were given the combined treatment experienced more incontinence (about 30% versus about 15 %), and naturally experienced more hormonal-ablation side effects such as hot flashes (in about 60% of the men).

Overall, then, there are still a lot of unknowns with hormonal ablation used in conjunction with radiation. But it does seem to be a promising option, so it's worth discussing with your doctor.

Cryosurgery

The technique of freezing the prostate and surrounding tissues has been used for many years in treating localized prostate cancer. Some time ago, this procedure had fairly severe side effects. Damage to the urethra and fistulas (openings of the urethra into the rectum) were not uncommon, and bladder-neck blockage was also a problem. Over the past few years, however, cryosurgery has improved quite a bit. We now have a better understanding of how the cancer should be frozen, better probes for freezing, transrectal ultrasound to guide doctors during treatment, and even a warming device that can be used during the procedure to help prevent damage to the urethra. These developments have helped reduce side effects, although impotence is still a common result of cryosurgery because the neurovascular bundles—where cancer is likely to spread—are usually frozen along with other areas.

In some cases, your doctor may want to use hormonal ablation therapy before cryosurgery. The idea is that the hormone therapy may shrink the prostate, thereby increasing the possibility that it can be completely frozen and reducing the risk of injury to the rectum, bladder and/or urethral sphincter. Also, hormonal therapy may enhance the destruction of tumor cells.

Cryotherapy, though, is generally considered to be a therapy for localized prostate cancer. It is not designed to treat disease outside of the prostate. (Just as a radical prostatectomy is not.) That is why radiation therapy is still considered to be the standard of care for patients with known T3 or T4 disease.

Neutron and proton radiation

Early results from research seem to support the use of neutron radiation in combating locally advanced cancer, and side effects from neutron radiation seem to be about the same as those resulting from traditional radiation.

Some institutions have started to look at using regular radiation and neutron radiation together, with impressive early results. For example, at Wayne State University in Detroit, Michigan, doctors using a combination of neutron and traditional photon radiation have found that four years after treatment, there was no evidence of disease in:

> ► 92% of the patients with an initial PSA of less than 10.
> ► 85% of the patients with an initial PSA of 10-20.
> ► 38% of those patients with an initial PSA greater than 20.

It is also interesting to note that those patients who received hormonal therapy before radiation treatment were on average 30% more likely to be disease-free after four years.

Overall, neutron radiation shows considerable promise, but more research is needed, and few places offer such treatments. As for proton radiation, the data for men with locally advanced disease receiving such treatments is very limited right now, in part because most studies have focused on localized prostate cancer.

Seed Implantation

Seed implants usually aren't used in T3 patients unless external beam radiation is also used. This is because doctors want to kill the cancer that has extended beyond the prostate, and seed implants are only effective against cancers within the prostate.

Also, if you are a candidate for seed implants, you and your doctor may want to discuss the use of hormonal ablation along with this procedure—again with the idea that this may work better if your prostate has been decreased in size.

Surgery

Fewer than 10% of urologists choose surgery as a treatment for locally advanced prostate cancer, and many believe it has no place in such cases. The problem with surgery in locally advanced cancer is that:

- ▶ it may not remove all of the cancer.
- ▶ there are potential complications with any surgical procedure, including a radical prostatectomy.
- ▶ there are good alternatives to surgery (as mentioned earlier).

Also, surgery in such cases requires the removal of more tissue than surgery for localized cancer requires. As a result, there is an increased risk of side effects, such as rectal injury and incontinence, and a much greater risk of erectile dysfunction.

There are a few situations where surgery may be the treatment of choice: For example, in some cases, the prostate may be removed in order to reduce most of the tumor (also called "debulking of the tumor"). This may allow the patient to live longer. Many doctors who perform surgery for locally advanced cancer do so in conjunction with hormonal therapy and/or radiation therapy .

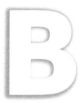

How Can Doctors Find and Treat Regionally Advanced Prostate Cancer (N1 Disease)?

Cancer of the lymph nodes is known by a number of names, including:

► D+ or D1 disease
► Local lymph node positive disease
► Lymphatic metastases
► Lymph node positive disease
► Lymphatic spread
► Nodal positive
► Node positive disease
► N+ disease which can also be classified as N1, N2, or N3
► Pelvic lymph node metastases
► Pelvic lymph node positive
► Regionally advanced prostate cancer
► Regional lymph node positive disease

Regionally advanced cancer—also known as nodal disease or N1 disease—involves the lymph nodes. Lymph nodes are everywhere in the body, but prostate cancer usually moves to nearby nodes first, much like a wave from a pebble moving outward across a pond. The first nodes to be affected by prostate cancer are usually those in the pelvic area, near the prostate. The next set of nodes typically affected are the abdominal lymph nodes, which lie in the area of the stomach and intestines. And the set of nodes usually affected after that are called the Peri Hilar/Supraclavicular Nodes, which lie in the chest, near the lungs and shoulders.

The older staging system divided nodal disease into three types, based on the size of the node. The newer system recognizes just one type of nodal disease: N1, or cancer that has metastasized or spread to one or more regional lymph nodes. (M1a is the new name for cancer that has gone to distant lymph nodes.)

In the past, 20% to 40% of the men diagnosed with prostate cancer had positive lymph nodes, but this number seems to have dropped to around 6% to 10%. This is a good sign, but because the total number of men who are diagnosed with prostate cancer has increased, there are more men today with cancer in the lymph nodes than ever before. If even just 6% of the 200,000 men diagnosed annually have node-positive disease, that means some 12,000 men will have regionally advanced disease.

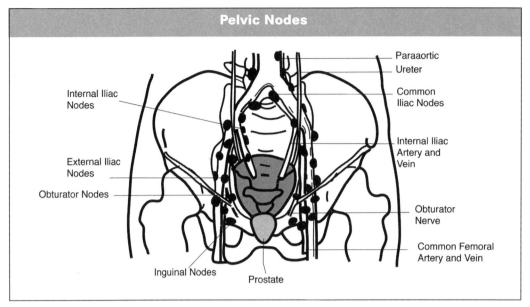

Pelvic Nodes

Paraaortic
Ureter
Common Iliac Nodes
Internal Iliac Nodes
Internal Iliac Artery and Vein
External Iliac Nodes
Obturator Nodes
Obturator Nerve
Common Femoral Artery and Vein
Inguinal Nodes
Prostate

The pelvic lymph nodes of the human body are the first set of nodes where prostate cancer usually goes after growing beyond the prostate area.

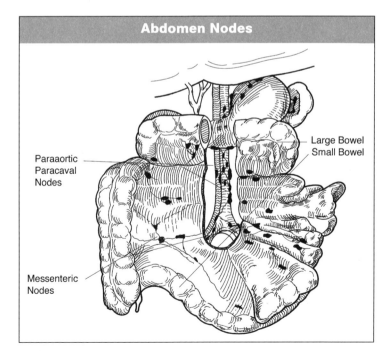

Abdomen Nodes

Paraaortic Paracaval Nodes
Large Bowel
Small Bowel
Messenteric Nodes

The abdominal pelvic lymph nodes of the human body are the second set of nodes where prostate cancer usually goes after growing beyond the prostate area.

Peri Hilar / Supraclavicular Nodes

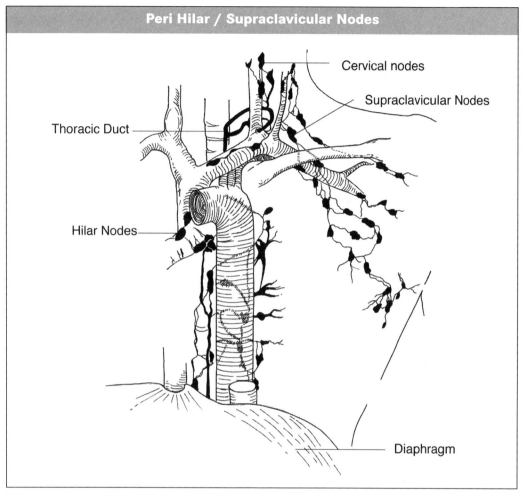

The Peri Hilar/Supraclavicular lymph nodes of the human body are the last set of nodes where prostate cancer usually goes after growing beyond the prostate area.

To diagnose regionally advanced disease, doctors will typically use some combination of the following tests:

▶ Biopsy

of the prostate to make the diagnosis.

▶ Bone Scan (for future comparisons)

to rule out bone metastases.

▶ CT Scan

to actually look for the lymph nodes.

▶ DRE

as part of the screening exam.

▶ Laparoscopic Pelvic Lymphadenectomy

used uncommonly to help decide on whether a patient has localized disease versus N1 disease.

▶ Monoclonal Antibody Imaging

rarely used at the time of initial diagnosis, but now commonly used in the face of disease recurrence to determine if cancer is present in the lymph nodes.

▶ MRI

occasionally replaces a CT scan.

▶ Physical Exam

rarely, prostate cancer spreads to the lymph nodes in the groin area and a doctor can feel cancer there because they are enlarged.

▶ PSA

the higher the PSA at diagnosis, the more likely that the cancer has spread to the lymph nodes.

▶ Transrectal Ultrasound (TRUS)

part of the original diagnostic tests, usually associated with the biopsy. Here it is not specific for detecting cancer that has spread to the lymph nodes.

Treatment Options for Regionally Advanced Cancer

Hormonal ablation

This is the most commonly used treatment for regionally advanced prostate cancer. There is some question about the best time to use this approach, however. That is, if cancer has spread to your lymph nodes, should you receive hormonal ablation right away, or should you wait until a later time when the cancer has spread farther?

That may sound odd, but some doctors think that waiting is worthwhile because hormonal ablation works for an average of two to three years before a person becomes "hormone refractory," or insensitive to hormone treatment. The

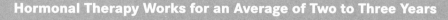

Hormonal Therapy Works for an Average of Two to Three Years

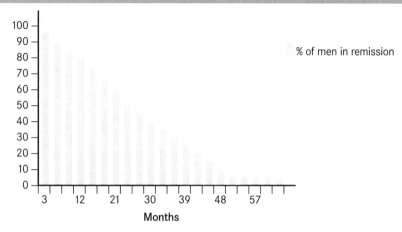

% of men in remission

Months

reasoning here is that by waiting, or at least using hormonal ablation intermittently, you still have it as a weapon against the cancer down the road.

At this point, no one can say which approach is best. We do know that early hormonal ablation may slow the progression of your cancer initially, but whether this translates into a longer survival time is not known. More research is underway, so discuss these options with your doctor. As you do, focus on quantity and quality of life with these treatments—it will help you decide what is best for you.

Radiation

The five- and ten-year disease-free survival rates for radiation of pelvic nodal disease are in the neighborhood of 7% to 33%—not especially good. Most studies seem to indicate that radiation to the lymph nodes provides little to no benefit, compared to no treatment at all.

The other key question that remains to be answered is whether or not patients who are at risk of nodal disease should get radiation beyond the prostate area to prevent cancer from spreading to the nodes. Studies that are now underway should help answer that question.

There is little or no data on the use of neutron or proton radiation for patients with node positive cancer. This will obviously change in the next few years, but right now any type of radiation for this stage is controversial. Again, if this is something you are considering, ask the doctor who would perform the treatment about his or her specific results, and about the side effects associated with the dosage of radiation in question.

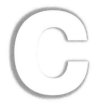

How Can Doctors Find and Treat Advanced Prostate Cancer (D2 or M1 Disease)?

Advanced prostate cancer is known as D2 or M1 disease, distant metastasis, metastatic prostate cancer, and nonregional prostate cancer, among other names.

At least 20 out of every 100 men diagnosed with prostate cancer have M1 disease. And this number does not take into account the thousands of men a year whose cancer progresses from a localized to an advanced stage. Any way you look at it, this is a serious problem.

Under the old staging system, M1 or D2 cancers were those that had spread far beyond the prostate or local lymph nodes (to the bones, liver, or lungs, for example). The newer staging system recognizes three types of M1 cancers:

► M1a. Cancers that have grown beyond the prostate and are now in nonregional lymph nodes, such as those near the lungs.
► M1b. Cancers that have gone to the bone(s).
► M1c. Cancer that is now in some other site(s) of the body, such as the liver, lungs, or other organs.

Diagnosing advanced prostate cancer

To diagnose advanced prostate cancer, doctors will typically use some combination of the following tests:

► Alkaline Phosphatase
to look for evidence of bone destruction by prostate cancer.
► Biopsy
(to confirm diagnosis).

▶ Bone Scan

to look for evidence of cancer spread to the bone.

▶ CT Scan

The CT scan is good at seeing changes in the organs, such as the liver and in the bones, caused by prostate cancer metastatses.

▶ Hemoglobin

a decrease in the Hb can be secondary to the fact that prostate cancer has spread to the bones.

▶ LDH

another chemical test that may indicate that prostate cancer is growing.

▶ Monoclonal Antibody Imaging

(for nonregional lymph nodes, or M1a) as described in previous chapters, this is a good test for looking for lymph nodes that are involved by prostate cancer.

▶ MRI

may be used instead of a CT scan.

▶ PAP

an enzyme that may be elevated in patients with metastatic disease.

▶ Physical Exam

doctors will be looking for pain on palpation of your bones as well as for lymph node enlargement.

▶ PSA

as discussed previously, the higher the PSA, the more likely it is that you will have metastatic disease.

▶ X-ray

can be used to look for cancer in the bones and can help distinguish between cancer and arthritis.

Treatment options for advanced cancer

The treatments for advanced cancer include hormonal ablation and chemotherapy. These treatments are discussed in more detail in the following chapters.

7

Hormonal Therapy

In this chapter:

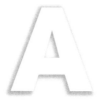

Why and When Should I Begin Hormonal Therapy?

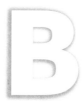

What Is Combined Hormonal Therapy?

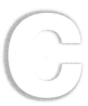

What Are the Newer Approaches to Hormonal Therapy?

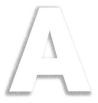

Why and When Should I Begin Hormonal Therapy?

When doctors refer to "hormonal ablation" what they are actually referring to is testosterone ablation or castration therapy. Testosterone is also known as a type of hormone called an androgen, and therefore these therapies can be referred to as antiandrogen therapies or androgen ablation. Although the names are different, the goal is to eliminate testosterone from the body. Today, hormonal ablation is used to treat prostate cancer patients at all stages of the disease, but it is usually given to patients with either locally advanced, regionally advanced, or metastatic cancer. Hormonal ablation is not used as a cure for prostate cancer. There are some cases in which men show no signs of cancer after hormonal ablation, but it is most often used to control the disease and provide relief from symptoms.

In men, the primary hormone is testosterone, which plays a role in everything from the production of sperm, the deepening of the voice, and the growth or loss of hair. Understanding how testosterone is made will help you understand hormonal therapy. In the brain, there is a structure called the hypothalamus which makes a hormone called "Luteinizing Hormone Releasing Hormone" (LHRH). LHRH travels from the hypothalamus to the anterior pituitary, which is also in the brain, to create "Luteinizing Hormone" (LH). This LH then travels down to the testicles, where it causes cells to make testosterone. The testicles make about 95% of the testosterone. The remaining 5% is produced from the breakdown of other steroids that are made from the adrenal glands.

Many prostate cancer cells need testosterone to grow, so doctors use hormonal therapy to try to stop the production of testosterone. For example, a patient might receive regular injections of LHRH agonist, a synthetic version of LHRH. This causes the body to "think" that there is too much LHRH in the system, and to become desensitized to the hormone. In essence, this means that the body begins to ignore LHRH; the anterior pituitary no longer recognizes it, and so it stops releasing LH, which in turn causes the testicles to stop making testosterone. (When a course of LHRH agonist injections begins, there is actually a large initial

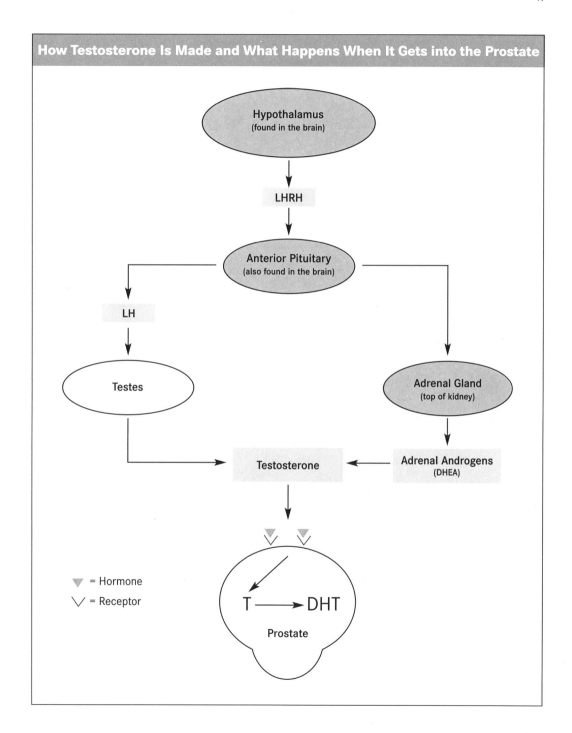

How Testosterone Is Made and What Happens When It Gets into the Prostate

Hypothalamus
(found in the brain)

LHRH

Anterior Pituitary
(also found in the brain)

LH

Testes

Adrenal Gland
(top of kidney)

Adrenal Androgens
(DHEA)

Testosterone

▼ = Hormone
∨ = Receptor

T ⟶ DHT

Prostate

increase in testosterone production, but after several weeks, desensitization takes effect and the testosterone production drops.)

Hormone (testosterone) levels are controlled using several methods:

► Surgical castration or "orchiectomy." This is a procedure in which the testicles are removed. Afterward, the production of testosterone stops almost immediately—or at least most of it does. About 5% to 10% of the body's testosterone is actually made in the adrenal glands, located on the top of the kidneys. This is one of the original treatments for advanced prostate cancer since it was a known treatment long before the LHRH agonists were developed. It is an inexpensive and effective form of androgen ablation; however, it does have drawbacks. First, it may be psychologically hard for a man to lose his testicles. Second, surgical castration removes the option of newer potential therapies such as intermittent androgen blockade, where men are cycled on and off LHRH therapy (see below). On the positive side, men do not have to be bothered by regular injections of the LHRH agonists and the treatment works equally well as the injection therapies.

► Medical castration, which involves injection with the LHRH agonists, as described above. LHRH is given through two types of injection: The Lupron injection, which is usually given in the buttocks, and the Zoladex injection which is usually injected in the abdomen. These injections only take seconds, and they both work about the same. A new medication, Abarelix, is being developed as an LHRH antagonist. This drug will not require antiandrogens to block the "flare response" (see page 132).

LHRH injections can be given every month, every three months, or every four months, depending on what you and your doctor are most comfortable with. The longer-lasting injections are certainly more convenient, but some health professionals feel that such long intervals tend to limit personal interaction between doctor and patient.

► Antiandrogen therapy. Inside the body, circulating testosterone enters prostate cancer cells and binds to 'androgen receptors.' Androgen receptors are then activated and allow the cells to grow. The antiandrogen drugs bicalutamide, flutamide, and nilutamide block, in part, circulating testosterone from binding to the androgen receptors. These drugs are not considered effective as single agents and, if used, are administered in combination with the LHRH agonists. These drugs do not allow the testosterone from the adrenal glands to reach the androgen receptor.

▶ Combined Hormonal Therapy (CHT), which involves the combined use of surgical or medical castration and an antiandrogen to decrease hormone levels. (This is discussed in more detail later in this chapter.)

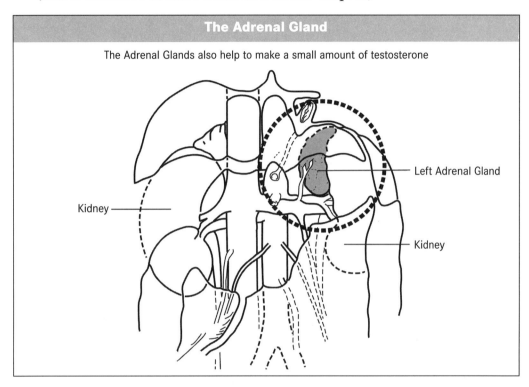

The Adrenal Gland

The Adrenal Glands also help to make a small amount of testosterone

Kidney

Left Adrenal Gland

Kidney

What happens when we reduce the levels of testosterone in the blood? Normally, the prostate cancer tumor shrinks and the PSA level decreases. The PSA decreases in over 90% of patients and will often become undetectable.

There are also side effects to consider. As you might expect, most of them are related to the decrease of male hormone levels. These side effects include:

▶ Loss of libido or sex drive (almost all patients)
▶ Impotence (almost all patients)
▶ Hot flashes (50% to 60% of patients)
▶ Sweating (10-15% of patients)
▶ Decrease in body hair (men need to shave less often)
▶ Fatigue (approximately 50% of patients)
▶ Weight gain (especially around the midsection) (almost all men)

In addition, patients on LHRH therapy sometimes experience "tumor flare," a condition in which testosterone increases 140% to 170% of its average level. This can be a "clinical flare" (with symptoms such as bone pain, urinary problems, or spinal cord compression), or a "biochemical flare" (with a rise in PSA). Tumor flare can be controlled with the use of an antiandrogen before or during LHRH therapy.

When is hormonal ablation used?

Hormonal ablation is sometimes used by itself for patients who have undergone watchful waiting; however, the use of it for patients with locally advanced (or suspected to be locally advanced) cancer is occurring more and more. That is, it can be given in the neoadjuvant setting (prior to the start of treatment), the concurrent setting (during treatment), and the adjuvant setting (after treatment). Finally, it is the first-line treatment for patients with advanced or metastatic prostate cancer.

Hormonal ablation and surgery

Hormonal ablation is sometimes given prior to surgery (neoadjuvant therapy) to try to reduce the size of the cancer in order to make it easier to remove, or in order to stop it from growing beyond the immediate area of the prostate. It is most likely to be recommended for men who have a high risk of having positive surgical margins—those with stage T2b or higher disease, PSA levels greater than 10-20, and a high Gleason score.

In general, studies have found a consistent decrease in prostate size and PSA with neoadjuvant therapy and surgery. Prostate size was reduced anywhere from 40% to 90%, and in virtually all the studies, 100% of the patients had a decrease in PSA. In addition, most trials have shown a significantly lower number of positive surgical margins—about a 10% to 30% decrease—in patients having neoadjuvant therapy versus those having only surgery.

There are, of course, drawbacks to this approach. Patients are on hormonal therapy for anywhere between three and eight months prior to surgery. Some experts believe that this may give the hormone resistant cells that may be present in the cancer more time to grow. In addition, some reports suggest that it can actually make surgery more difficult, because the prostate experiences a type of scarring or fibrosis reaction that makes it difficult to identify the prostate margins and to cleanly cut the prostate out. In addition, we are not sure right now if hormones given during surgery are effective.

Hormonal ablation and radiation

Hormonal ablation is sometimes used with radiation because it may reduce the number of cells that need to be destroyed by radiation, and it may make cancer cells more vulnerable (see Chapter 6).

Neoadjuvant and concurrent therapy

A study done in the 1970s using DES (an estrogen) prior to radiation therapy for locally advanced cancers showed an almost 20% higher rate of local control, compared to radiation therapy alone. Other studies using other hormones before and during radiation therapy found 25% better control rates for cancer than radiation therapy alone.

However, the best length of time to use hormonal therapy in conjunction with radiation is not yet known. Some studies are now extending neoadjuvant therapy from three months to eight months before therapy, and the early findings seem to suggest improved results for patients undergoing the longer therapy. Most of these studies keep the patient on hormone ablation while the radiation is given.

Concurrent and adjuvant therapy

In 1998, a study showed that men with T3 and T4 prostate cancer may keep cancer away longer and live longer if they are given hormonal ablation as soon as radiation is started, and then for three years after treatment. In this study:

▶ about 80% of the men receiving combined treatment were alive five years after treatment, versus a little more than 60% of the men receiving only radiation.
▶ of the patients who were alive after five years, 85% had no signs of disease, versus 48% of those who received radiation alone.

This appeared to be great news for men with locally advanced prostate cancer, but more research is needed if we are to be certain. Also, there are some things to remember when considering those results. For example:

▶ The men in the study were either given radiation or radiation with hormonal ablation. There were no patients in the study who received hormonal ablation alone. It could be that patients would do just as well on hormonal ablation with no other treatment.
▶ The study only followed patients for about four years—the rest of the data was based on estimates.
▶ Men who were given the combined treatment experienced more incontinence (about 30% versus about 15%), and naturally experienced more hormonal-ablation side effects such as hot flashes (in about 60% of the men).

Overall, there are still a lot of unknowns with hormonal ablation used in conjunction with radiation. But it does seem to be a promising option, so it's worth discussing with your doctor.

Hormonal ablation and cryotherapy

At this point, there is still much to learn about the use of hormonal ablation with cryotherapy. Neoadjuvant therapy before cryotherapy is sometimes offered to patients with large prostates (greater than 40 grams) or locally advanced cancers. The goal is to shrink the prostate, which increases the chance of completely freezing the cancerous tissue, while reducing the risk of injuring the bladder, rectum and urethral sphincter. It may also cause apoptosis—or "cell death"—in hormone-sensitive prostate cancers. However, any long-range benefit from neoadjuvant therapy with cryotherapy has not been proven.

Hormonal ablation and advanced disease

Hormonal ablation is the first therapy used when a patient has advanced or metastatic prostate cancer. It is very effective in controlling the cancer and usually decreases the PSA to undetectable. It is also very effective at controlling pain for patients who have metastases to bones. Hormone therapy in the patient with advanced disease works for an average of 2-3 years before this therapy starts to become ineffective. In some people, however, hormone therapy works for many years.

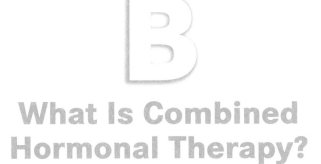

What Is Combined
Hormonal Therapy?

As we mentioned before, not all of the androgens made in a man's body come from the testicles. A small but significant amount comes from the adrenal glands. Although many doctors are satisfied with the results of medical or surgical castration, some believe that an antiandrogen should also be given to eliminate the testosterone and other androgens produced by the adrenal glands. This approach is called Combined Hormonal Therapy (CHT) or Maximal Androgen Blockade

(MAB). Proponents of this combined approach think that CHT may:

- ▶ provide a better initial response by preventing tumor flare.
- ▶ delay the development of more hormone-insensitive prostate cancer cells.
- ▶ slow the progression of prostate cancer.
- ▶ increase survival.

Unfortunately, none of these things has been proven. Monotherapy (single drug therapy with Lupron or Zolodex) and CHT can both be considered standards of care for patients with metastatic disease. Some doctors use monotherapy, and others use CHT. It is a matter of doctor and patient preference. What is known is that an antiandrogen should initially be used in combination with an LHRH agonist to prevent a flare response. A flare response can occur because in the first few weeks of use the LHRH agonists can actually increase the amount of testosterone in the body which could fuel the prostate cancer to grow. This is only a temporary problem and the antiandrogen can be stopped after the first month if the patient is going to continue on monotherapy.

They are two types of antiandrogens: pure antiandrogens and steroidal antiandrogens.

Pure antiandrogens block the binding of testosterone to its receptor. They are most commonly used in combination with LHRH agonists or surgical castration. It is rare to use them alone as a first option treatment for advanced disease. The pure antiandrogens include:

▶ Flutamide (trade name, Eulexin)

One of the more commonly used antiandrogens, flutamide is used in men with metastatic prostate cancer as initial therapy; in combination with medical or surgical castration; or when metastatic prostate cancer does not respond to medical or surgical castration. It is an oral drug that is given two to three times per day. Some of the side effects are:

Hot flashes (in approximately 60% of patients)
Diarrhea (in approximately 10% of patients)
Breast enlargement, or "gynecomastia" (in approximately 10% of patients—this can be avoided by treating the area with radiation beforehand)
Liver problems (in approximately 5 - 10% of patients)

▶ Bicalutamide (trade name, Casodex)

A commonly used antiandrogen which is newer than Flutamide. It appears to be as effective as the commonly used Flutamide, and carries with it a lower chance of having diarrhea. It is an oral drug taken only once per day. Side effects include:

    Hot flashes (in 40% of patients)
    Nausea (in 10% of patients)
    Nipple tenderness (in 5% of patients)
    Itching (in 5% of patients)
    Breast enlargement, or "gynecomastia" (in 5% of patients)

▶ Nilutamide (trade name, Nilandron)

Another one of the newer antiandrogens. Side effects include:

    Hot flashes (in 25% - 30% of patients)
    Impaired vision in the dark (in 10% - 15% of patients)
    Nausea (in 10% of patients)
    Constipation (in 5% - 10% of patients)
    Dizziness (in 5% -10% of patients)
    Lung inflammation, or pneumonitis (in 1% - 5% of patients)

Steroidal antiandrogens, such as Cyproterone Acetate (also known as CPA), are not used in the United States, but doctors do prescribe them in Europe, Canada, and other parts of the world.

Triple androgen blockade

Another therapy that a few physicians have started to use is called triple androgen blockade. In this therapy, Finasteride (Proscar) is added to CHT. Finasteride is the drug that blocks the conversion of testosterone to its more active breakdown product, dihydrotestosterone. Currently, there is no clear evidence that this is an effective treatment for hormone-sensitive prostate cancer.

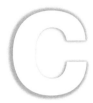

What Are the Newer Approaches to Hormonal Therapy?

Immediate versus delayed hormone therapy: The case of the patient with the rising PSA.

It is now becoming increasingly common that the only symptom in a patient with advanced disease is a rising PSA. (This is most frequently seen in a man who was treated for localized disease and the bone scan and the CT scan are still negative.) Alternatively, hormonal therapy may have cleared previously seen prostate cancer from bone scans or CT scans.

As we have said, doctors' understanding of prostate cancer is growing, and new approaches and tools are continuing to evolve. One area that is still being explored is the timing of treatment for advanced prostate cancer. That is, is it best to give hormonal ablation immediately after diagnosis, or to wait until the individual actually shows symptoms of the disease?

When patients hear of this discussion, they usually ask "Why would I want to delay treatment?" The argument for delaying is that if a patient has no symptoms of advanced disease, hormonal treatment will produce significant side effects at a time when they would otherwise feel good.

The argument against delayed treatment is more obvious. A rising PSA means that the prostate cancer will eventually surface somewhere (most likely in the bones) and even if immediate treatment does not lead to better survival rates, delaying might increase the likelihood of problems with the bladder, urination, kidneys, and bones (for example, spinal cord compression).

Unfortunately, for patients with PSA-only disease we do not know what the best answer is. Some doctors believe we should start treatment right away, others when the PSA reaches a specific number (10, 20, 50....), and still others favor waiting until there is either clinical or scan evidence of disease. You should consult with your doctor and discuss which decision is best for you.

Immediate versus delayed hormone therapy: The case of clinically evident or scan-positive disease.

The situation of when to treat appears to be clearer here. The results from a large study started in 1985 indicate that progression of the prostate cancer is more likely to be slowed by immediate treatment. In this study, patients with M0 disease and delayed treatment developed metastatic cancer faster, bone pain occurred earlier, and overall progression or advancement of disease was faster. Also, more of these men needed TURPs (30% of delayed-treatment patients vs. 14% of immediate-treatment patients). However, the authors of the study could not make an absolute recommendation applicable to all men with prostate cancer. The study is still going on, and we should know more in a few years. However, there is some good evidence even now to start hormonal therapy early in this situation. Ultimately, the decision about how to proceed is up to you and your doctor, so you should both be armed with as much information as possible about ongoing studies in this area.

Intermittent Therapy—a new form of hormonal therapy

Some doctors believe that hormone therapy may at times encourage the growth of hormone-insensitive and aggressive prostate cancer cells. Based on some laboratory studies that supported this idea and the knowledge that hormonal therapy has side effects, a study was done that demonstrated that patients on intermittent therapy had a similar survival and an increased quality of life as compared to patients on continuous hormonal therapy. To really know if this type of therapy is better, a study that directly compares the two therapies needs to be completed. While it is being conducted currently, the results will not be known for several years. Therefore, intermittent therapy is still considered experimental. Although there are no absolute guidelines, intermittent therapy is usually administered by starting a patient on CHT for approximately 6-8 months, until the PSA is undetectable. The patient is then taken off CHT and his testosterone is allowed to rise. This allows the hormone-sensitive cells to start to grow again. This will, of course, allow the PSA to start to rise. When the PSA reaches a point decided upon by the doctor, the CHT is restarted and the cycle continues. Although we do not know if this therapy increases survival, it does appear to increase quality of life, and doctors are using this treatment more and more.

Sequential Therapy—another new form of hormonal therapy

This approach uses a combination of Finasteride (Proscar—the drug that blocks the conversion of testosterone to its stronger metabolite, dihydrotestosterone [DHT]) and a receptor-blocking antiandrogen (such as Flutamide or Bicalutamide)

Intermittent Hormonal Therapy

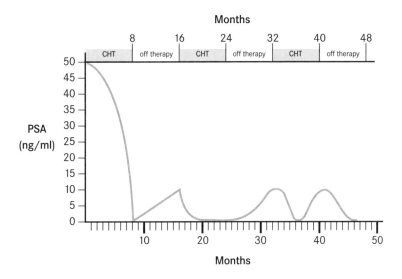

to treat prostate cancer without reducing testosterone levels. It is called "sequential" because the two establish a kind of sequence of defense. The receptor-blocking antiandrogen stops testosterone from binding to the androgen receptor; if some androgen gets through, the Finasteride prevents it from being converted to DHT.

This approach does not seem to be as effective as castration in treating prostate cancer. The main advantage is that patients may be able to treat their cancer while maintaining high testosterone levels, which means fewer side effects in terms of reduced sexual desire and function. The quality of life of these patients is very high but it is unknown how well this treatment really works. It remains experimental.

Second-Line Hormonal Treatments

If you are on hormonal ablation, but your cancer continues to progress, one of your options is second-line hormonal treatment. The data in this area are severely limited, but are growing rapidly. Below are some of the second-line options.

The addition of an antiandrogen if you are on monotherapy

Occasionally, if a man on monotherapy experiences a rising PSA, his doctor will add an antiandrogen to his therapy. This slows the progression of the disease temporarily in approximately 10% of patients. Although this seems like a low number, it may be worth trying for a patient with no symptoms.

Surgical castration if medical castration is not working

A question commonly asked by patients is whether they should have a surgical castration if the drugs are no longer working. This is actually simple to answer. If your physician checks your testosterone and it is at "castrate" level, then there is no need for surgery. This is the case almost all of the time.

Antiandrogen Withdrawal Syndrome—the first step in patients on hormonal therapy with CHT

Sometimes, the peripheral antiandrogens can actually begin to make the cancer grow after patients take them for awhile. This appears to be due to the presence of altered or mutated androgen receptors that begin seeing the antiandrogen as an androgen. Therefore, when a rising PSA is seen in patients on CHT, the first step is to stop the antiandrogen (Flutamide, Bicalutamide, Nilutamide). This works to decrease the progression of the cancer in 10%-30% of patients for an average of three to eight months. In addition, this syndrome can be observed with any hormonal treatment, so most doctors look for it if you have been taking any of the second-line treatments listed below.

Estrogens

Some patients are surprised that estrogen can be used for the treatment of prostate cancer, but this is not a new concept. Estrogens have been used a great deal in men (and still are). We know that estrogens go to the brain and decrease the amount of LH that is released. They may also be involved in the actual killing of cancer cells. Initially there were cardiovascular problems associated with its use, but these can usually be minimized by using smaller dosages. A commonly used estrogen is DES (diethylstilbestrol).

DES as a second-line hormone given at 1 mg/day was effective in decreasing the PSA in 40% of patients for an average of 8 months. DES appears to be a good option for patients who have failed or are failing LHRH therapy. Estrogens are inexpensive ($5 - $15 dollars a month) and work as well as common hormonal ablation, but they fell out of favor years ago because they were associated with slightly more side effects. As a result, DES is difficult to find in the United States. Finally, if you are on estrogen you might also need to be on a blood-thinning drug (Coumadin or Warfarin) or aspirin in order to reduce your chances of developing blood clots.

▶ Ketoconazole (trade name, Nizoral)

This drug blocks the production of testicular and adrenal androgens. It may also kill prostate cancer cells directly (as shown in the lab). The average dose is high—400 mg three times a day— and is associated with a large number of gastrointestinal problems. Objective responses of 15% and stable disease have been reported in about 30% of patients. Stable disease means the cancer does not shrink or that the PSA does not go down, but stays where it is for awhile. Ketoconazole is usually given with a steroid to replace the steroids that are no longer produced by the adrenal gland. More recently, this drug and hydrocortisone were used in men whose cancer progressed after experiencing Flutamide withdrawal—the antiandrogen withdrawal described earlier in this chapter. Out of 48 patients:

▶ 45% - 50% had a greater-than 80% PSA decrease for about four months.
▶ 60% - 65% had a greater-than 50% PSA decrease for about four months.

▶ Glucocorticoids (steroids)

Glucocorticoids prevent adrenal testosterone production. The three glucocorticoids most commonly used in treating prostate cancer are:

▶ Prednisone, which in one study was found to decrease pain in about 40% of patients, and about 20% demonstrated a decrease in PSA for an average response of four months (but the range was 3 to 30 months).
▶ Hydrocortisone, which has led to a subjective response in about 60% of patients.
▶ Dexamethasone, which also has led to a subjective response in about 60% of patients.

▶ High-Dose Bicalutamide (trade name, Casodex)

In a study of 10 patients with progressive metastatic prostate cancer who had failed CHT, four (or 40%) of the men felt better after therapy. One man who did not respond also had a large increase in pain and PSA, which went away when the Bicalutamide was stopped.

Another study looked at 52 men with advanced prostate cancer who showed disease progression following medical or surgical castration. There was no objective response seen, but almost a third of the patients had stable disease and their self-pain score went down within three months after taking Bicalutamide. In addition, the average man survived about 15 months.

A recent study has demonstrated that 150 mg daily of Casodex appears to be as effective as treatment with an LHRH agonist.

In summary, there are several treatments that your doctor may want to discuss with you if first-line medical or surgical castration fail.

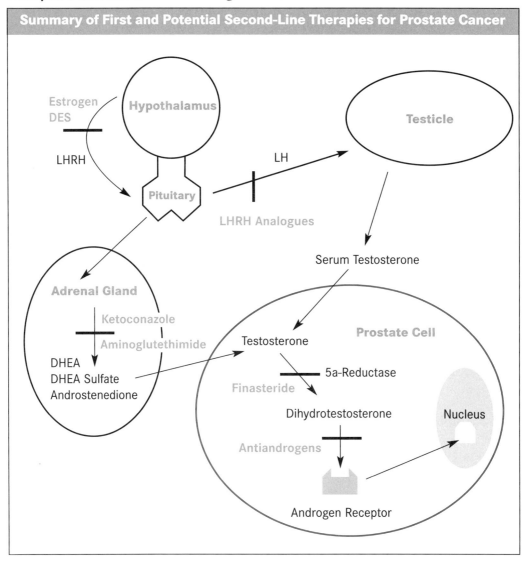

Summary of First and Potential Second-Line Therapies for Prostate Cancer

8

Beyond Hormonal Therapy: Next Steps

In this chapter:

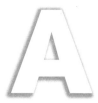

What Are the Standard Chemotherapy Options and When Should They Be Used?

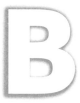

What Are the Newer Chemotherapy Combinations and Treatments?

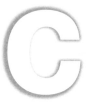

Farther Out: What Kind of Treatments Are Being Explored by Scientists?

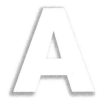

What Are the Standard Chemotherapy Options and When Should They Be Used?

As mentioned earlier, radiation therapy and surgery are most effective in treating localized prostate cancer, or in simply slowing advanced cancer. Hormonal therapy is more often used for advanced cancer, but it is useful for only a limited time, because people become "hormone-refractory," or insensitive to such therapy, after about two to three years, on average. At that point, doctors turn to chemotherapy to fight the cancer.

PSA and Advanced Disease

Since 1992, PSA has been used to measure the response of advanced prostate cancer to various treatments. Several studies and trials have shown a direct relationship between decreases in PSA and shrinkage of measurable prostate tumors as well as increased survival for patients who decreased their PSA by greater than 50% from their baseline value.

A special note on the use of PSA and advanced prostate cancer: In localized disease, we can use a PSA of 4 as an upper limit of normal to screen for cancer—but this is not the case with androgen-independent cancers. Each tumor creates a unique amount of PSA, which is relative to each individual. That means each patient has his own unique starting point, or baseline; a patient may have a small amount of cancer and a high PSA, or a large amount of cancer and a low PSA.

So remember: It is essentially meaningless to compare your PSA to that of another patient. There are patients who have a PSA of less than 10 who have many bone metastases and need narcotics to control their pain. Other patients with PSAs over 1,000 have no pain. There is no magic PSA number that correlates with symptoms or death! The important thing is whether your PSA number goes up or down, because that generally (but not always) correlates with whether your cancer is growing or shrinking.

Chemotherapy refers to the use of drugs that attack and kill cancer cells. There are many different types of chemotherapy drugs that kill cancer cells in different ways. Some attach themselves to the DNA and do not allow it to copy itself. Others stop the cancer cells from dividing. All chemotherapy drugs work by killing cells that are dividing. Cancer cells grow faster than normal cells in the body and that is why chemotherapy works. It is also why people who take chemotherapy often lose their hair—because it, too, is growing rapidly and the chemotherapy drugs kill the hair cells temporarily.

For many years, chemotherapeutic drugs for hormone refractory prostate cancer were used and analyzed as single agents given alone and in combination with other drugs, with poor results. In general, the average survival rate in these studies has been something like six to nine months. Over the last five years, multiple new effective drugs and regimens have become available and survival and quality of life of men with hormone-refractory disease is increasing. We can see the progress almost monthly! We have seen men live many years after being diagnosed with hormone-refractory disease. Results of chemotherapy can vary widely. It really comes down to looking at each individual patient and how he is going to be treated for his hormone-refractory prostate cancer.

At present, there are only a few standard approaches to treating hormone-refractory patients. However, the National Comprehensive Cancer Network (NCCN), an organization of cancer centers around the country, has reviewed all of the studies that have been done recently in hormone-refractory disease and has set guidelines for care. In other words, these are regimens that experts in the field of prostate cancer feel can make a difference in the quantity and quality of life of patients with hormone-refractory disease. These therapies are all new in the last five years and more are coming. Again, the drugs were chosen based on demonstrated anticancer activity and acceptable toxicity. The combinations include:

Ketoconazole (Nizoral) and Doxorubicin (Adriamycin)

In a study of this combination, a PSA decrease of more than 50% was seen in 55% of patients. About 29% of the patients developed complications such as acral erythema (redness of the hands and feet) and stomatitis (mouth sores). However, once Doxorubicin was stopped, the symptoms disappeared. When a symptom went away, the Doxorubicin was resumed and the symptoms did not return. The overall NCCN statistics for this combination are:

▶ Response Rate:

(the response rate tells you how many patients respond to a given treatment—usually this correlates with living longer)

  ▶ PSA Response in 55% of patients (doctors define a PSA response as a >50% decrease in PSA from baseline that is held for at least 4 weeks)

  ▶ Soft Tissue Response in 60% of patients (a soft tissue response is measured in two ways: a partial response [PR] is a 50% decrease in the size of a measurable mass [usually a lymph node on a CT scan], or a complete response [CR], which is complete disappearance of the lesion).

▶ Side Effects:

  ▶ A few patients (two) died suddenly from treatment

  ▶ Stomatitis and acral erythema: 30% of patients

  ▶ Serious anal mucositis in 13% of patients (sloughing of the inner lining of the lower gastrointestinal tract—this causes very painful bowel movements, diarrhea, and bleeding temporarily)

Vinblastine (Velban) and Estramustine (Emyct)

The combination of Vinblastine and Estramustine seems to enhance tumor killing in preclinical models of prostate cancer. In trials, PSA decreases of more than 50% were found in 54% to 61% of the patients. This therapy was well tolerated—meaning it produced relatively few side effects. One trial showed that patients who experienced a greater than 50% decline in PSA had significantly increased overall and progression-free survival. The overall NCCN statistics for this combination are:

▶ Response Rate:

  ▶ PSA Response in 55%-60% of patients

  ▶ Soft Tissue Response in 15%-40% of patients

▶ Side Effects:

  ▶ Nausea in 20% of patients

  ▶ Leukopenia (decrease in white blood cells in 12% of patients)

  ▶ Constipation in 20% of patients

  ▶ Transient neuropathy in 12% of patients (neuropathy is a condition that causes patients to experience numbness and tingling in their hands and feet)

Etoposide (VePesid) and Estramustine

In laboratory tests, the combination of Etoposide and Estramustine has been shown to kill cancer cells and impair the replication of DNA by the cancer cell.

In a trial, a PSA decrease of greater than 50% was demonstrated in 55% of patients. Estramustine caused significant nausea in about 30% of patients. Other trials that used a lower dose of Estramustine showed a PSA decrease of greater than 50% in about 40% of the patients, with less nausea. If you are using this combination of drugs, your doctor will probably want you to take the Estramustine with food and avoid calcium-rich products—such as milk, yogurt, ice cream, antacids containing calcium, etc.—which can interfere with the absorption of the drugs. The overall NCCN statistics for this combination are:

▶ Response Rate:
    ▶ PSA Response in 40% - 60% of patients
    ▶ Soft Tissue Response in 45% -55% of patients

▶ Side Effects:
    ▶ Nausea
    ▶ Hair loss (also known as "alopecia")
    ▶ Leukopenia (decrease in white blood cells in 25% of patients)
    ▶ Blockage of the veins ("Deep Vein Thrombosis" or "DVT" in approximately 10% of patients)

Mitoxantrone (Novantrone) and Prednisone

This combination of drugs has focused on decreasing pain for patients with hormone-refractory prostate cancer. In many studies using this combination, a high percentage of patients experienced a complete response or partial response, meaning they had:

▶ a 50% decrease in pain medication (analgesic) use with no increase in pain
▶ a decrease of 2 points on a 6-point pain scale, with no increase in analgesic use

Serious side effects were limited to leukopenia (a decrease in the number of white blood cells that fight infection).

Because of these studies, the combination of Mitoxantrone/Prednisone as a treatment for hormone-refractory prostate cancer has been approved by the Food and Drug Administration as a way to control pain in patients with hormone-refractory prostate cancer. The overall NCCN statistics for this combination are:

▶ Response Rate:
    ▶ PSA Response in 33% of patients

▶ Palliative Response (relief/comfort) in approximately 30%-50% of patients

▶ Side Effects:
   ▶ A small amount of nausea
   ▶ Leukopenia (decrease in white blood cells in 5 - 10% of patients)

Paclitaxel (Taxol) and Estramustine

Paclitaxel and Estramustine have been shown to inhibit the way cancer cells divide. In one study looking at this combination, a PSA decrease of more than 50% was achieved in 53% of patients. The combination is now being tested using a variety of dosage schedules, and early results seem promising. The overall NCCN statistics for this combination are:

▶ Response Rate:
   ▶ PSA Response in 53% of patients
   ▶ Soft Tissue Response in 44% of patients

▶ Side Effects:
   ▶ Nausea
   ▶ Breast enlargement (also known as "gynecomastia")
   ▶ Fluid retention
   ▶ Leukopenia (decrease in white blood cells in 20% of patients)

Continued Androgen Suppression

A controversial area in the treatment of androgen-independent prostate cancer has been whether a patient who is going to take chemotherapy for hormone-refractory prostate cancer should stay on hormone therapy. In the past, most patients with metastatic prostate cancer were treated with surgical castration either as first-line treatment or at the time of failure of hormone therapy via injections. Most patients enrolling in clinical trials for androgen-independent disease still had received some form of androgen ablation. With the widespread availability of medical forms of reversible hormone therapy using LHRH agonists (Lupron or Zoladex) and/or antiandrogens, the question of the role of continued hormone therapy in hormone-refractory disease has become important. A retrospective review of patients enrolled in chemotherapy trials for androgen independent disease tried to answer this question. It was concluded that continued hormone therapy was not a significant factor in patient survival. However, another review showed a modest survival advantage for patients with continued hormone therapy. Also, many patients feel more secure remaining on hormone therapy. At this time, it is the general consensus of oncologists (cancer specialists) to keep patients on hormone therapy while we evaluate new therapies for hormone-refractory prostate cancer. This way, all of the patients who receive chemotherapy can be compared in a similar fashion.

What Are the Newer Chemotherapy Combinations and Treatments?

A number of drugs and drug combinations for advanced prostate cancer are still being tested, and have not yet been approved or endorsed by the government or any national organization. Some of these are listed below. We provide this list because some patients with hormone-refractory prostate cancer may want to find out more about them, and keep track of developments in these areas.

Estramustine and Docetaxel (Taxotere)

The combination of Estramustine and Docetaxel has been demonstrated to be very effective at killing prostate cancer cells in preclinical models. In a recent study using this combination, 63% percent of the patients had a drop in their PSA of greater than 50%, and a number of patients were able to discontinue their use of pain medication. The results of multiple Phase II studies are beginning to be available. (A Phase II study tests a specific regimen of drugs in a specific disease to find out the response rate.) Overall, the statistics for this combination are:

- ▶ Response Rate:
    - ▶ PSA response in 80-90% of patients
    - ▶ Soft tissue response in 75% of patients

▶ Side Effects:
  ▶ Edema: swelling in the legs
  ▶ Fatigue
  ▶ Esophagitis: inflammation of the esophagus that can be painful and make it temporarily difficult to eat

Estramustine, Etoposide, and Paclitaxel

This combination was tested because of the activity of Estramustine and Etoposide together and the activity of Estramustine and Paclitaxel together. Overall, the statistics for this combination are:

▶ Response Rate:
  ▶ PSA Response in 53% of patients
  ▶ Soft Tissue Response in 40% of patients

▶ Side Effects:
  ▶ Nausea
  ▶ Hair loss (also known as "alopecia")
  ▶ Fatigue
  ▶ Leukopenia (decrease in white blood cells in 10 - 20% of patients)

Although these statistics do not seem as good as the two drug combination, the side effects were less with the three drug combination. Also, many of the patients the regimen was given to had received other chemotherapy regimens first, and this generally lowers the response rate.

Cyclophosphamide (Cytoxan), Diethylstilbestrol (DES), and Prednisone

In a test of this combination, doctors looked at a group of patients that had previously failed combined hormone therapy and had evidence of a rising PSA following antiandrogen withdrawal. Almost 40% of these patients showed a decrease in PSA of more than 50%. This triple combination was well tolerated by patients. Overall, the statistics for this combination are:

▶ Response Rate:
  ▶ PSA Response in 40% of patients
  ▶ Soft Tissue Response in 33% of patients

▶ Side Effects: Minimal

Doxorubicin and Ketoconazole, alternating with Vinblastine and Estramustine

This regimen has been tested extensively at the M.D. Anderson Cancer Center in Houston. The regimen is a bit difficult to follow because the treatment covers 56 days (more than twice as long as most other treatments), with each of the various drugs being given on certain days in the cycle. Side effects have been manageable. Overall, the statistics for this combination are:

▶ Response Rate:
  ▶ PSA Response in 67% of patients
  ▶ Soft Tissue Response in 75% of patients

▶ Side Effects:
  ▶ Edema or swelling in 50% of patients
  ▶ Deep Vein Thrombosis in 18% of patients (A deep venous thrombosis [DVT] is a blood clot in the veins of the leg. This leads to swelling of the leg and the patient then needs to be treated with a blood thinner such as coumadin, generally for 6 months)
  ▶ Cardiac problems in 4% of patients

Suramin

Suramin is part of a new class of drugs that inhibit growth factors (these drugs are called growth-factor antagonists). In the laboratory, it has also been shown to inhibit enzymes that help DNA to grow and replicate, and to slow growth in some prostate cancer cell lines. One of the problems with Suramin is that it can cause nerve damage at high dosages. Newer dosing guidelines and schedules that do not require heavy monitoring were developed and tested, making it more feasible to conduct trials; however, it is not being actively developed at this time.

Using the Immune System: Vaccines, Antibodies and Gene Therapy

One of the things that make treating cancer difficult is that the disease can hide from the immune system. The immune system consists of white blood cells (WBC) in the body that recognize foreign substances or cells and destroy them. WBCs are also called leukocytes. They use the lymph nodes as their home bases to go out and fight infection. One type of WBC is called the neutrophil and it fights bacterial infections. Another kind of white blood cell, the lymphocytes, fights infection caused by viruses and destroys other cells, such as cancer cells, that are bad for the body. This is accomplished in one of two ways:

▶ A subset of lymphocytes, the T cells, helps destroy cancer cells directly.

▶ A second type of lymphocyte, the B cell, produces antibodies when it comes across a foreign cell. These antibodies attach to the cancer cell and tell another set of WBCs, the macrophages, that a bad cell is present, and come to help destroy it.

Since T and B cells do not seem to recognize cancer very well, several researchers are trying to find and develop prostate cancer-specific antigens, or proteins, that will mark the cancer cells more effectively. They then inject these antigens under the skin and hope the immune system will recognize them as foreign and mount a response to them. This type of therapy is called a vaccine. Multiple vaccine trials are underway in the United States. In general, they are targeted at men with a rising PSA after failing local therapy such as a prostatectomy or prostatectomy + radiation. Some vaccine trials are open for men with hormone-refractory disease. Results from vaccine trials so far have been mixed. On the negative side, they only seem to help a small percentage of patients. On the positive side, they have virtually no side effects. Vaccine trials, in general, open and close very quickly and it is difficult to predict which ones will be available at a given time. The good news is that means doctors are developing better and better strategies to test all of the time.

Another approach is gene therapy, which is already available in several forms. Here, a gene is inserted into some of the lymphocytes, which changes them into far more effective cancer fighters. An alternate procedure inserts a gene that makes the cells "super attractors" for other cancer-fighting cells. These types of trials are still rare and it is more likely that various vaccine strategies will be used to unmask the immune system to fight the cancer over the next several years.

Another way to use the immune system is to use antibodies. Cancer cells do express specific antigens or proteins on their cell surface that mark them as foreign to our bodies or specific to the cell type (like prostate specific membrane antigen [PSMA]). Several researchers are trying to isolate those antigens. When they do, they then make an antibody to it, which is another protein that binds to the antigen. The next part of the strategy is to attach a "radioactive bomb" to the antibody (such as radioactive iodine) and inject that into the patient. These antibodies will then "hone into" the cancer and destroy it with radioactivity. Antibody trials are still fairly rare, but should become more available over the next few years.

Radiation Therapy:

Radiation is a very effective way to treat painful metastases from metastatic prostate. This can be done in two forms, as local therapy or as systemic therapy with an agent such as Strontium-89.

Local therapy (or spot radiation) can be used to treat painful bone metastases at a single site. In general, the radiation is given as 10 treatments (of 300 'rads' each) over a two week period. Pain relief is achieved in the vast majority of patients. It can occur rapidly, but sometimes takes up to a month to see good results.

Systemic radiation therapy is given in the form of an injection into the blood of Strontium-89, a radioactive isotope. It is used for patients with multiple sites of pain from bone metastases. It hones into where bone is being hurt and kills the cancer cells nearby. Multiple studies have demonstrated that it provides at least partial relief in 60% to 80% of patients and lasts approximately 6 months. One potential side effect of Strontium-89 is that it can lower your platelet count and can sometimes interfere with the future use of chemotherapy. Therefore, we prefer to try to use chemotherapy to control hormone-refractory prostate cancer before using Strontium-89.

Antiangiogenesis Therapy:

New tumors often need blood to grow, so researchers hope that by reducing the growth of blood vessels feeding a tumor, they can reduce or stop its growth. Preclinical laboratory tests show much promise in this area, using the drugs Angiostatin and Endostatin. These drugs started in Phase 1 clinical trials in September 1999. Phase I trials are open to all patients and look for the toxicity of a drug and to establish the proper dosage. After doses are established, specific trials in prostate cancer will be started. There are other possible antiangiogenesis agents that are also in clinical trials but it is too early to determine if they will be effective in the treatment of hormone-refractory prostate cancer. The best thing to do is ask your doctor or to check the National Cancer Institute's Clinical Trials Web site which lists current trials than are ongoing.

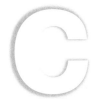

Farther Out: What Kind of Treatments Are Being Explored by Scientists ?

Antisense therapy

Cancer is associated with the faulty production or performance of proteins that tell the cell how to grow and what to do. With antisense therapy, researchers use synthetic segments of DNA or RNA to stop the production of such disease-related proteins. This method involves the use of antisense compounds—that is, compounds that make no genetic sense—to block the transmission of genetic information going from the nucleus to the protein-production sites in the cell, which halts the production of the faulty proteins. Clinical trials of this approach should begin soon.

Blocking signal transduction

Signal transduction pathways are the chemical routes that transmit messages through the cell's cytoplasm to its nucleus. Many of the cancer-related genes (oncogenes) that scientists have identified appear to be abnormal versions of signaling pathway components. Many scientists are trying to develop drugs and therapies that will block abnormal signal transduction pathways associated with cancer.

Antimetastasis therapy

As you no doubt know by now, metastasis is the process by which cancer cells spread from a primary tumor to other sites in the body. For a cell to successfully move from the primary tumor, several steps need to take place. The cell needs to walk away from the primary tumor, enter the bloodstream, survive circulating through the bloodstream, stop at the place it wants to establish itself, then dig into that tissue. Then it grows into a metastasis. Researchers are trying to block several steps in this pathway. Marimastat is a drug that stops the cancer cell from breaking down the environment around the primary tumor so that it cannot walk out.

It currently is in clinical trials. Another possibility is modified citrus pectin, a drug that blocks the circulating cancer cell from stopping or adhering to the metastatic site. This drug is also in clinical trials.

Looking ahead

This is an exciting time in the development of new therapies for the treatment of advanced prostate cancer, and there are many clinical trials of advanced prostate cancers being conducted today. These include trials sponsored by the National Cancer Institute (NCI) and drug companies. A good place to find clinical trials is at Cancer Centers. Another source on the Internet is the NCI's trials list. The address is: http://207.121.187.155NCI_Cancer_Trials/. There are many sites on the World Wide Web dedicated to prostate cancer—some of which advertise clinical trials. Patient support groups can also be a good source of information about such trials. (See support groups and other helpful organizations, page 174.)

9

Dealing with Cancer Pain and Other Symptoms

In this chapter:

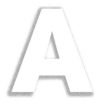

What Are Some of the Treatments for Cancer Pain?

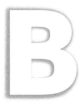

What Are Some of the Other Problems that I Should Be Aware of?

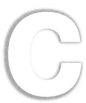

What Are Some of the Alternative Approaches to Dealing with Symptoms and Problems?

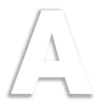

What Are Some of the Treatments for Cancer Pain?

An important part of dealing with advanced prostate cancer treatment is palliative care, which is essentially any therapy that comforts the patient and relieves symptoms of the disease. Hormone ablation and chemotherapy are considered effective forms of palliative therapy in advanced prostate cancer, but there are several other treatments and drugs that may be called upon as needed.

Radiotherapy for Bone Pain

The majority of prostate patients with hormone-refractory disease have problems because their cancer has typically spread to the bones, where it can cause pain due to bone damage, bone fractures, and pressure on the bones from the expansion of the cancer. Pain can occur for a short time or it can be continuous, and the site of pain may move and change depending on your activity or even changes in the weather.

External beam radiation therapy in the form of local or "spot" radiation can be effective in controlling such symptoms in a specific area. For example, if you have pain in one spot on your spine, then radiation can be given to that specific area to kill the cancer and relieve the pain. This is usually given in the form of 10 treatments of radiation in the space of approximately two weeks.

Nearly 80% of patients with bone pain will experience at least partial pain relief with radiation treatment, and about 40% of patients will have total pain relief. Side effects are relatively minor, and often depend on the site being treated. For example, radiation to the upper abdomen can cause nausea and vomiting, while radiation to the upper spine can lead to a sore throat or difficulty in swallowing. Such temporary symptoms can usually be treated with medications.

Strontium-89 (Metastron)

Another approach that has been the subject of much research is the use of injectable radiation or radioisotopes. One of these, Strontium-89, has been particularly well studied. Strontium-89 is effective because it follows the same path as calcium into the bones, but rather than settle into normal healthy bone, it goes to areas where the bone is changing—which tends to be the cancerous area. Studies of Strontium-89 therapy show that:

▶ About 80% of patients have pain relief with this type of therapy—typically, in one to two weeks.

▶ In the 80% of patients who respond to Strontium-89, the effect lasts about three to eight months—at which time another dose can be given.

▶ About 50% of patients can expect to decrease their use of painkillers with this treatment. Strontium-89 can be given safely to patients who have been previously treated with radiotherapy for relief of symptoms.

▶ Patients treated with Strontium-89 in combination with radiotherapy had a significantly lower rate of developing new painful bone lesions, and those who developed new lesions had fewer of them.

▶ If the first injection is not helpful, then chances are others will not be helpful either.

If you have kidney problems, you need to be monitored carefully when receiving this treatment, because the Strontium-89 is, of course, radioactive, and excreted through the kidneys. For the same reason, patients need to double-flush the toilet after urinating to make sure the slight amounts of radioactive material are taken away. The greatest potential side effect of Strontium therapy, however, is a reduction in the number of platelets, which aid in clotting the blood. So as a rule, we generally give Strontium only after we have tried chemotherapy.

Evaluating Pain

Individual patients have very different thresholds of pain. There are several pain scales used to evaluate pain, but the simplest method asks you to rate your pain on a scale of 1 to 10. This gives your doctor a reference point for tracking changes in your perception of pain over time.

Aspirin and Acetaminophen (Tylenol)

Aspirin and Tylenol are probably the most common pain medicines used. However, they are not very effective in treating bone pain related to prostate cancer.

Nonsteroidal Antiinflammatory Drugs (NSAIDs)

These drugs are considered to be the first-line therapy for bone pain associated with prostate cancer. In reaction to the presence of cancer in your body, the immune system tries to fight it by sending various white blood cells to the area where cancer is present. These white blood cells gather to fight the cancer directly (by attaching to them and killing them) as well as indirectly (by releasing chemicals called cytokines that attract other cells). This gathering of cells around the cancer is called inflammation. NSAIDs can help in treating bone pain because they stop the inflammation associated with your cancer. They are primarily used for milder pain, and patients who experience bone pain for the first time can be effectively treated with NSAIDs such as Ibuprofen. Patients react differently to medications, you may need to try more than one to find which one works best for you. Your doctor may also want you to take an "H2-blocker" which are forms of antacids to help prevent any stomach upset from the NSAIDs.

Some of the commonly used NSAIDs are:

▶ Voltaren Diflunisal
▶ Dolobid
▶ Advil, Motrin, Nuprin
▶ Indocin
▶ Toradol
▶ Orudis
▶ Relafen
▶ Naprosyn
▶ Alleve
▶ Feldene
▶ Clinoril
▶ Tolectin

Narcotics

Narcotics are strong antipain medicines that work by blocking pathways in the brain that mediate pain called opiate receptors. They are used in addition to the NSAIDs. Many narcotics can be given either orally or via injection; one, known as Fentanyl, can also be delivered through a patch worn by the patient. There are many different doses and forms of narcotics. They are available in weak and strong forms as well as short-and long-acting doses.

Commonly used narcotics include:

▶ Morphine

- Codeine
- Fentanyl
- Percodan
- Dilaudid
- Methadone

Steroids

Steroids are another form of antiinflammatory drugs. They are also an effective therapy to treat bone pain. They work in a manner similar to NSAIDs; however, they can be associated with more side effects such as water retention and suppression of your ability to fight infection. At lose dose, however, they are very safe. Different doctors use steroids at different times for the treatment of bone pain.

Commonly used steroids include:

- Cortisone
- Dexamethasone
- Hydrocortisone
- Methylpredisolone
- Prednisone

Bisphosphonates

Some men with advanced prostate cancer may experience bone-pain relief from the use of diphosphonates (also called bisphosphonates). Bisphosphonates fight the breakdown of bone, and there are several trials underway to see if these drugs are effective in blocking the spread of prostate cancer as well as in treating painful bone metastases.

Commonly used bisphosphonates:

- Ibandronate
- Etidronate
- Clodronate
- Pamidronate
- Zolendronate

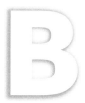

What Are Some of the Other Problems that I Should Be Aware of?

Anorexia/Cachexia

Anorexia and cachexia—weight loss, lack of appetite, and a general decrease in body function—affect as many as 60% to 70% of patients with advanced prostate cancer. Nutritional supplements can be used to help in such cases, as can high-calorie, high-nutrition meals. Steroids have also been found to stimulate appetite, but they do not usually lead to long-term improvement. In addition, megesterol acetate (Megace) has been demonstrated to stimulate appetite in some patients.

Back Pain

When a patient with advanced prostate cancer has back pain, it should be treated as an emergency. This is because back pain is the primary symptom in 90% of patients who experience spinal-cord compression. The spinal cord runs down the middle of your back, protected by your spine, and carries the nerves from your brain to the rest of your body. Spinal cord compression afflicts about 10% of patients who have hormone-refractory disease. Patients who have back pain or who have numbness or tingling running down a leg should be treated with steroids as soon as possible. If the spinal cord is blocked, radiation or surgery will usually be used to provide relief.

Urinary Obstruction/Hematuria

If the prostate or the cancer spreads to the bladder, it can lead to urinary obstruction and blood in the urine (hematuria). If the patient is unable to urinate, urinary catheterization is usually used as a short-term solution. A TURP may be performed as a longer-term solution.

Blood in the urine (which can be caused by radiation as well as cancer) can clot in the urinary tract. To treat it, catheterization might be used, or your doctor

163

may rely on certain agents, such as silver nitrate, alum, and ethamsylatea, to decrease the bleeding. Sometimes sources of bleeding can be found in the bladder or along the urinary tract that can be cauterized to stop clots from forming.

Fluid Retention

Sometimes when the cancer spreads to the lymph nodes deep in your body, it can partially block the return of blood to the heart. This causes the water part of the blood to leave the veins in the legs and move into the lower part of the legs, causing swelling. In addition to treating the cancer to shrink the lymph nodes we often try to remove the water using diuretic medicines. These medicines increase the amount you urinate which helps move the water out of your legs.

Constipation

Opiate drugs can cause constipation because they slow the natural movement of the bowels. Men with advanced cancer may also be less likely to move around, or drink or eat adequately, which also contributes to constipation. To avoid and treat constipation, it's helpful to drink eight glasses of water a day and stay active. Also:

> ► Laxatives, such as Milk of Magnesia, Citrate of Magnesia and, polyethylene glycol-electrolyte solutions can be helpful.
> ► Other laxatives, such as Metamucil, can also be useful but should be taken with caution—if you don't drink enough water when using these laxatives, the situation can get worse, and the feces can become impacted.
> ► Surfactant laxatives such as dioctyl sodium sulfosuccinate should also be used with caution because they depend on bowel movement, and if you are on narcotic drugs, that movement is inhibited.
> ► Stimulant laxatives such as senna and cascara, and anthraquone laxatives such as Senokot, must be used carefully because they are very strong. These typically work within 24 hours, and are preferred in many cases.
> ► Lubricants such as mineral oil are useful for chronic constipation.

Finally, suppositories and enemas can be effective, but they are usually used only after other options have been exhausted. How to best treat constipation in each person varies dramatically. It is best that when you start on a narcotic pain medicine, you also go on a propylactic regimen to prevent constipation at the start—ask your doctor what might be best. Also, don't wait to treat constipation; in general, it only gets worse!

Anemia

Anemia—a lack of red blood cells—is often seen in advanced prostate cancer patients because the cancer can affect the cell-producing areas of the bones. Anemia can also be a side effect of radiation or chemotherapy. Symptoms of anemia include:

- ▶ shortness of breath
- ▶ chest pain (angina)
- ▶ fatigue
- ▶ lack of overall energy
- ▶ confusion

If you have serious anemia, your doctor may give you a blood transfusion. Transfusions don't help every patient. If you have had one in the past and it has not helped, chances are that another won't help either. Talk to your doctor to find out what is likely to work in your situation.

Another possibility is to take something called erythropoietin (also called "Procrit"), which can stimulate the production of blood cells. However, this can be expensive and is not always effective, so transfusions are usually tried first.

Depression

About 25% of the men who have advanced prostate disease experience significant depression—and many are afraid to admit it! It is very important that you help your doctor recognize that you may be depressed. It makes it harder to treat your cancer. Some common symptoms of depression are difficulty sleeping, lack of appetite, fatigue, loss of will to do any activity, and loss of enjoyment in any activities. If you are experiencing these symptoms you can see why they will only make worse how you might be feeling due to your cancer! Some of the common antidepressants used to treat this condition are:

Type of Antidepressant	Name
Tricyclic antidepressant	Amitriptyline (Elavil)
	Doxepin (Sinequan)
	Imipramine (Tofranil)
	Nortriptyline (Pamelor)
Selective serotonin reuptake inhibitors (SSRI)	Fluoxetine (Prozac)
	Paroxetine (Paxil)
	Sertraline (Zoloft)
	Venlafaxine (Effexor)

Tricyclic antidepressants take two to four weeks to really work, and some of them may aggravate problems with urination. SSRI drugs usually work faster, and have fewer urinary side effects than the tricyclic drugs. Also, some over-the-counter herbs seem to help in cases of mild depression (see the discussion of St. John's Wort, in section C of this chapter).

In addition to taking such medications, you might find it useful to consult a therapist. This is true for spouses and other family members, too, because they may be having emotional difficulties during your illness.

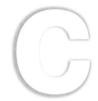

What Are Some of the Alternative Approaches to Dealing with Symptoms and Problems?

Many alternative or complementary approaches have been tried for the treatment of prostate cancer. Many of these approaches involve supplements, which are called "supplements" because they are just that—supplements or additions to the diet.

Kava Kava and Anxiety

Not surprisingly, some men experience a great deal of anxiety when they are diagnosed with prostate cancer. The supplement Kava Kava (kavalactones) may be helpful in such cases. Clinical trials have used a range of 100 mg to 200 mg of kavalactones daily in divided doses, or as a single dose at bedtime. Long-term use of higher doses (400 mg of kavalactones) can result in some scaling of the skin on the legs and arms. If you are thinking about using Kava Kava, talk to your doctor.

St. John's Wort and Depression

The herb St. John's Wort (Hypericum perforatum) can be considered in cases of mild to moderate depression. Research suggests that its effectiveness in such cases is comparable to that of conventional drug treatment.

The safest approach is to buy a St. John's Wort supplement that contains at least 0.3% hypericin (the active ingredient). The usual dosage is 300 mg to 900 mg per day (given in divided daily doses). St. John's Wort seems to have relatively mild side effects compared to conventional antidepressants. However, you may experience sensitivity to light; gastrointestinal upset; dizziness; restlessness; and constipation. There is also some concern about potential interactions with other antidepressants. You should consult your doctor before starting another antidepressant if you are taking St. John's Wort.

Acupuncture and Pain/Nausea

Acupuncture is sometimes used to treat chronic pain and nausea in advanced prostate cancer patients, and a number of studies suggest that such treatments can be effective. Acupuncture costs are sometimes covered by health insurance; even if they aren't, our experience indicates that the out-of-pocket expense for the treatment is relatively low—perhaps $50 to $100 dollars per treatment.

There are some cautions. For example:

► The research on acupuncture involving placebo groups is limited, and there is no research on acupuncture for advanced prostate cancer.
► Side effects such as infection and bleeding are possible, especially if you are treated by an acupuncturist who has not received adequate training. With a well-trained acupuncturist, however, side effects from this procedure are few.
► Patients have to evaluate for themselves whether a practitioner has had adequate training in acupuncture. Many states do not require acupuncturists to have specific training—just an M.D. or D.O. degree.

Overall, we think that acupuncture can be helpful in treating cancer pain and nausea that is a result of chemotherapy, but we don't think it should be used as a complete substitute for more conventional options.

Meditation and Stress Reduction

Meditation can reduce stress and help you to be mentally prepared for coping with treatments and situations in your life. One study showed that individuals who meditate produce greater amounts of melatonin, a substance that some researchers think may have cancer-fighting properties. There are plenty of classes and books on meditation that are available. We think it is worth at least looking into, especially if you are feeling a great deal of stress.

PC-SPES

PC-SPES is a commercially available supplement that is a combination of eight herbs. Available since late 1996, it has been used by many patients with prostate cancer. We have followed a number of patients who used it, and detected a decreased PSA within two to six weeks in some patients who had advanced disease. There are some side effects, including breast enlargement, that seem to increase with the dosage. Men taking this supplement should know that there is a possibility of venous thrombosis (clotting of the blood in the legs).

PC-SPES is fairly expensive, and there are significantly cheaper options. For example, DES and other estrogens cost perhaps $5 to $15 a month—as opposed to several hundred dollars for PC-SPES—and may work as well as PC-SPES. The bottom line is that no one is really sure how well either of these options work, so they should be discussed with your doctor.

A Note on Supplements

There are a number of supplements that may be helpful, or harmful, in fighting prostate cancer or treating its symptoms. (For a more detailed look at supplements, see *The ABCs of Nutrition & Supplements for Prostate Cancer*, by Mark Moyad, M.P.H., also published by Sleeping Bear Press. To order visit your local bookstore or call 1-800-487-2323.)

10

The Five Commandments for Getting the Most out of Your Visit to the Doctor

In this chapter:

Commandment I: Be Prepared

Commandment II: Bring Support

Commandment III: Ask Questions

Commandment IV: Take Notes

Commandment V: Have Realistic Expectations

The time you spend with your doctor is critically important, but it is also limited. These commandments will help you evaluate your situation and get information that will help you make decisions about how to proceed.

Commandment I: Be Prepared.

Often, doctors spend a lot of time explaining the basics to a patient, which can waste valuable time. The more time you invest in learning the basics on your own, the more time you will have to ask your doctor important questions, and the better your chances are of gaining new knowledge about your illness and possible treatments. It's that simple.

Before your next visit to the doctor, consider making preparations such as:

▶ Making a list of questions you want to ask.
▶ Updating your knowledge of tests and treatments.
▶ Familiarizing yourself with your medical records. You might also want to keep a personal health journal, and create a summary of PSA results (along with treatments) over the past year or two.
▶ Asking your doctor what you need to bring in on your next visit. For example, do you need to bring copies of your medical records and test results?
▶ Familiarizing yourself with your medical insurance so that you understand exactly what it covers. For example, does it pay for experimental treatments? What sort of deductible do you have?

Commandment II: Bring Support.

It's a good idea to bring along your wife or partner, a family member, or even a friend when you visit the doctor. The emotional and mental assistance this provides is invaluable—for both you and your partner. Also, it's not uncommon for a spouse to remember important details and questions during a visit. We know from research that spouses can be affected mentally and physically when their husbands are diagnosed with prostate cancer. Ask doctors and therapists how you can assist each other during this difficult time.

Commandment III: Ask Questions.

The best way to find out what you want to know is to ask questions. As we mentioned above, bring a list of the questions that are on your mind. It's important to focus on the most important questions, because surveys have shown that only about 25% of the questions brought in by patients are actually answered. So, it's a good idea to write down the top five or ten, rather than every question you can think of. For example, an important question might be, "What is your success rate with this treatment?" And a less important question might be, "How soon after the treatment can I play golf again?"

Never be afraid to tell your doctor what is on your mind, and never be afraid to ask an "embarrassing" question. It's your health that is being discussed in these visits, so don't be intimidated. Also, remember that questions that seem embarrassing to you are probably routine for the doctor. If your doctor doesn't want to give you the information you want, or seems to discourage questions, it might be time to find another doctor. Communication and mutual respect are important components of a good doctor-patient relationship.

Commandment IV: Take Notes.

Recalling all of the questions and answers that occurred during your visit is virtually impossible. Always bring a pad of paper and a pen to your visit (we recommend black ink, in case you want to photocopy your notes). If you are asking good questions and communicating well with your doctor, there will usually be a lot to remember, and writing things down can help you keep track. Another great idea is to take a tape recorder, so that you can listen to the tape as a reference for you and others.

Commandment V: Have Realistic Expectations.

You should always evaluate all the information you can gather before deciding on anything, carefully weighing the pros and cons of each course of action. The opinions of your doctors, spouse, support group members, books, and other sources are all parts of the total picture, and when you put them together you should be able to arrive at decisions that are right for you. You will also feel better knowing that you have evaluated and compared all of your options before making a decision. When it comes to advanced prostate cancer, the more sound opinions you get, the better. There is no single definitive treatment for this disease—instead, it usually involves a number of different treatments, and treatment possibilities are evolving and growing. So, don't take one person's advice or experience as the final word. Instead, consider getting opinions:

- ▶ from several doctors.
- ▶ from individuals who have been in a similar situation.
- ▶ from spouses who have watched their partner go through the treatment.
- ▶ from books, articles and the Internet.

Few things in life are perfect, and that's true of prostate cancer treatments. Every treatment has its good points and bad points. Insist on knowing all the pros and cons of treatments, and inquire about:

▶ Your likely financial cost.

▶ Potential side effects. That means not just general or overall side effects, but specifically those that can be expected when this doctor performs the procedure. Ask what percentage of the doctor's patients experience side effects and how long those side effects last. Also, ask the doctor to define the words being used. For example, if he or she says a side effect is impotence, does that mean temporary or permanent impotence? Complete or partial loss of erectile function? Words mean different things to different doctors.

▶ How are the side effects normally treated? Would a medication correct it? Does it usually go away with time? Would surgery be needed to correct it?

▶ What is your doctor's success rate with this treatment? How is success measured? By PSA? By other lab values? By months or years of living longer?

▶ If you are receiving a new kind of test, how accurate is it? What percentage of participants get false positives or false negatives? What conditions make it more likely to get a false reading? Is this the best time to have this test done?

▶ Does it decrease pain or improve mobility? Does it increase life expectancy?

▶ If you have other medical conditions, how does the treatment affect or interact with those conditions? For example, if you are experiencing early signs of osteoporosis, hormonal therapy could make the osteoporosis worse. If there is a potential problem, are there ways to minimize the risk?

▶ Can alternative treatments affect treatment? Can they be used in combination with conventional treatment?

▶ Is the treatment FDA approved or is it experimental? If it is experimental, why hasn't it been FDA approved?

Finally, be sure to question your doctor closely if he or she says a certain treatment or test is the only option. At nearly every stage of prostate cancer, there are many options to consider. Make sure your doctor is giving you a thorough, objective explanation of them all. These commandments will help you get the most out of your doctor's visits and at the same time will serve to empower you with the most knowledge about your cancer.

Support Groups and Other Helpful Organizations

There is a lot of help available for men with prostate cancer and their loved ones. Below is an alphabetical summary of major national organizations that can put you in touch with support groups and other resources in your area.

American Cancer Society (ACS)
1599 Clifton Road N.E.
Atlanta, GA 30329-4251
(800) ACS-2345

American Foundation for Urologic Disease (AFUD)
1128 North Charles Street
Baltimore, MD 21201
(410) 468-1800
(410) 468-1808 fax

Canadian Cancer Society
10 Alcorn Avenue - Suite 200
Toronto, Ontario, Canada M4V 3B1
Cancer Information Service toll-free (888) 939-3333
(416) 961-7223
(416) 961-4189 fax

Cancer Care Inc.
275 7th Avenue
New York, NY 10001
(800) 813-HOPE
(212) 302-2400
(212) 719-0263 fax

CaPCURE, Inc.
1250 Fourth Street - Suite 360
Santa Monica, CA 90401
(310) 458-2873
(301) 458-8074 fax

Choice in Dying
1035 30th Street N.W.
Washington, DC 20007

(800) 989-WILL
(202) 338-9790
(202) 338-0242 fax

Corporate Angel Network (CAN)

Westchester County Airport
One Loop Road
White Plains, NY 10604
(914) 328-1313
(914) 328-3938 fax

Education Center for Prostate Cancer Patients (ECPCP)

380 North Broadway - Suite 304
Jericho, NY 11753
(516) 942-5000
(516) 942-5025 fax

Matthews Foundation for Prostate Cancer Research

1142 Northeast 58th Street
Kirkland, WA 98033
(800) 234-6284
(425) 893-9657 fax

National Cancer Institute

9000 Rockville Pike
Bethesda, MD 20892
(800) 532-4440
(800) 4-CANCER (Cancer Information Service): A nationwide telephone service for cancer patients and their families, as well as the general public and health care professionals, that answers questions and provides free booklets about cancer.
(301) 402-5874 (CancerFax): Provides treatment summaries, with current data on prognosis, relevant staging and histologic classifications, news and announcements of important cancer-related issues.

National Hospice Organization (NHO)

1700 Diagonal Road - Suite 300
Alexandria, VA 22314
(800) 658-8898

National Prostate Cancer Coalition (NPCC)

1156 15th Street N.W. - Suite 905
Washington, DC 20005
(202) 463-9455
(202) 463-9456 fax

Patient Advocates for Advanced Cancer Treatments (PAACT)

1143 Parmalee N.W.
Grand Rapids, MI 49504
(616) 453-1477
(616) 453-1846 fax

Prostate Cancer Research & Education Foundation (PC-REF)

6699 Alvarado Road
Suite 2301
San Diego, CA 92120
(619) 287-8866

Prostate Cancer Resource Institute (PCRI)

5777 West Century Blvd. - Suite 885
Los Angeles, CA 90045
(310) 743-2110
(310) 743-2113 fax

U.S. Food and Drug Administration (FDA)

Drug Information Branch - HFD210
5600 Fishers Lane
Rockville, MD 20857
(301) 827-4573

US TOO International, Inc.

930 North York Road - Suite 50
Hinsdale, IL 60521-2993
(800) 808-7866
(630) 323-1002
(630) 323-1003 fax

Glossary & Index

Abdomen
the part of the body below the ribs and above the pelvic bone that contains organs like the intestines, liver, kidneys, stomach, bladder and the prostate

Ablation
reduction of; for example, in the management of prostate cancer, the killing off of cancer cells by radiation, cryotherapy, hormonal therapy, or chemotherapy

Adenocarinoma
a form of cancer that develops from a malignant abnormality in the cells lining a glandular organ such as the prostate; almost all prostate cancers are adenocarcinomas

Adjuvant
an additional treatment used to increase the effectiveness of the primary therapy; radiation therapy and hormonal therapy are often used as adjuvant treatments following a radical prostatectomy

Adrenal Glands
the two adrenal glands are located above the kidneys; they produce a variety of different hormones, including sex hormones-the adrenal androgens make about 10% of circulating testosterone

Adrenalectomy
the surgical removal of one or both adrenal glands

Adriamycin
A chemotherapy agent for advanced prostate cancer

Age-Adjusted
modified to take account of the age of an individual or group of individuals; for example, prostate cancer survival data and average normal PSA values can be adjusted according to the ages of groups of men

Alkaline Phosphatase
an enzyme in blood, bone, kidney, spleen and lungs; used to detect bone or liver metastasis

Alpha-Blockers
pharmaceuticals that act on the prostate by relaxing certain types of muscle tissue; these pharmaceuticals are often used in the treatment of BPH, but not in the treatment of cancer

Analog
a synthetic chemical, or pharmaceutical, that behaves very like a normal chemical in the body, e.g. LHRH analogs

Anandron
trade or brand name for Nilutamide, an antiandrogen

Androcur
trade name for cyproterone, an antiandrogen

Androgen
a hormone which is responsible for male characteristics and the development and function of male sexual organs (e.g., testosterone) produced mainly by the testicles but also in the cortex of the adrenal glands

Anesthetic
a drug that produces general or local loss of physical sensations, particularly pain; a "spinal" is the injection of a local anesthetic into the area surrounding the spinal cord

Aneuploid
having an abnormal number of sets of chromosomes; for example, tetraploid means having two paired sets of chromosomes, which is twice as many as normal

Angiogenesis
the formation of new blood vessels; a characteristic of tumors

Anterior
the front; for example the anterior of the prostate faces forward

Antiandrogen
a compound (usually a synthetic pharmaceutical) which blocks or otherwise interferes with the normal action of androgens at cellular receptor sites

Antiandrogen Withdrawal Response (AAWR)
a decrease in PSA caused by the withdrawal of an antiandrogen such as bicalutamide (Casodex) or Flutamide (Eulexin) or nilutamide (Anadron) after combined hormonal therapy (CHT) begins to fail; it occurs when there are PCa cells that have mutated to feed on the anti-androgen rather than testosterone (T) or dihydrotestosterone (DHT)

Antibiotic
a drug that can kill certain types of bacteria

Antibody
protein produced by the immune system as a defense against an invading or "foreign" material or substance (an antigen); for example, when you get a cold, your body produces antibodies to the cold virus

Anticoagulant
a drug that helps to stop the blood from clotting

Antigen
"foreign" material introduced into the body (a virus or bacterium, for example) or other material which the immune system considers to be "foreign" because it is not part of the body's normal biology (e.g., prostate cancer cells)

Anus
the opening of the rectum

Apex
the tip or bottom of prostate, e.g., the part of the prostate farthest away from the bladder

Aspiration
the use of suction to remove fluid or tissue, usually through a fine needle (e.g., aspiration biopsy)

Asymptomatic
having no recognizable symptoms of a particular disorder

Autologous
one's own; for example, autologous blood is a patient's own blood which is removed prior to surgery in case a patient needs a transfusion during or after surgery

Base
the base of the prostate is the wide part at the top of the prostate closest to the bladder

Benign
relatively harmless; not cancerous; not malignant

Benign Prostate Hyperplasia (or hypertrophy) (BPH)
a noncancerous condition of the prostate that results in the growth of both glandular and stromal (supporting connective) tissue, enlarging the prostate and obstructing urination

Benign Prostatic Hypertrophy (BPH)
similar to benign prostatic hyperplasia, but caused by an increase in the size of cells rather than the growth of more cells

Bicalutamide
a nonsteroidal antiandrogen available in the USA and some European countries for the treatment of prostate cancer; also known as Casodex

Bilateral
both sides; for example, a bilateral orchiectomy is a procedure in which both testicles are removed and a bilateral adrenalectomy is an operation in which both adrenal glands are removed

Biopsy
sampling of tissue from a particular part of the body (e.g., the prostate) in order to check for abnormalities such as cancer; in the case of prostate cancer, biopsies are usually carried out under ultrasound guidance using a specially designed device known as a prostate biopsy gun; removed tissue is typically examined miscroscopically by a pathologist in order to make a precise diagnosis of the patient's condition

Bladder
the hollow organ in which urine is collected and stored in the body

Blood Chemistry
measured concentrations of many chemicals in the blood; abnormal values can indicate spread of cancer or side effects of therapy

Blood Count
analysis of blood cells and platelets; abnormal values can indicate cancer in the bone or side effects of therapy

Bone Marrow
soft tissue in bone cavities that produces blood cells

Bone Scan
a technique more sensitive than conventional x-rays

which uses a radiolabeled agent to identify abnormal or cancerous growths within or attached to bone; in the case of prostate cancer, a bone scan is used to identify bony metastases which are definitive for cancer which has escaped from the prostate; metastases appear as "hot spots" on the film; however, the absence of "hot spots" does not prove the absence of tiny metastases. Bone scans can also be positive because of old injuries or arthritis

Bowel Preparation
the cleaning of the bowels or intestines which is normal prior to abdominal surgery such as radical prostatectomy

BPH
(see Benign Prostate Hyperplasia)

Brachytherapy
A form of radiation therapy in which radioactive seeds or pellets which emit radiation are implanted in order to kill surrounding tissue (e.g., the prostate, including prostate cancer cells)

CAB, Complete Androgen Blockade
(see CHT)

Cancer
the growth of abnormal cells in the body in an uncontrolled manner; unlike benign tumors, these tend to invade surrounding tissues and spread to distant sites of the body via the bloodstream and lymphatic system

Capsule
the fibrous tissue that acts as an outer lining of the prostate

Carcinoma
a form of cancer that originates in tissues which line or cover a particular organ; (see Adenocarcinoma)

Casodex
brand or trade name of bicalutamide

Castration
the use of surgical or medical techniques to eliminate testosterone produced by the testes

Cat Scan
Computerized Axial Tomography (also CT) is a method of combining images from multiple x-rays under the control of a computer to produce cross-sectional or three-dimensional pictures of the internal organs which can be used to identify abnormalities; the CAT scan can identify prostate enlargement, but is not always effective for assessing the stage of prostate cancer; for evaluating mestastases of the lymph nodes or more distant soft tissue sites, the CAT scan is significantly more accurate

Catheter
a hollow (usually flexible plastic) tube which can be used to drain fluids from or inject fluids into the body; in the case of prostate cancer, it is common for patients to have a transurethral catheter to drain urine for some time after treatment by surgery or some forms of radiation therapy

CDUS
color-flow Doppler ultrasound; an ultrasound method that more clearly images tumors by observing the Doppler shift in sound waves caused by the rapid flow of blood through tiny blood vessels that are characteristic of tumors

CGA, Chromagraphin A
a small cell prostate cancer or neuroendocrine cell marker

CHB, Combination Hormone Blockade
same as CHT or ADT (androgen deprivation therapy) or MAB (maximal androgen blockade) usually involving an LHRH agonist and an antiandrogen

Chemotherapy
the use of drugs or other chemicals to kill cancer cells

CHT, Combined Hormonal Therapy
the use of more than one hormone in therapy; especially the use of LHRH analogs (e.g., Lupron, Zoladex) to block the production of testosterone by the testes, plus antiandrogens, e.g.,Casodex (bicalutamide), Eulexin (flutamide), Anadron (nilutamide), Androcur (Cyproterone), to compete with DHT and T (testosterone) for cell sites, thereby depriving cancer cells of DHT and T needed for growth

Clinical Trial
a carefully planned experiment to evaluate a treatment or a medication (often a new drug) for an unproven use; Phase I trials are very preliminary short-term trials involving a few patients to see if drugs have any activity or any serious side effects; Phase II trials may involve 20 to 50 patients and are designed to estimate the most active dose of a new drug and determine its side effects; Phase III trials involve many patients and compare a new therapy against the current standard or best available therapy

Complication
an unexpected or unwanted effect of a treatment, drug, or other procedure

Conformational Therapy
the use of careful planning and delivery techniques designed to focus radiation on the areas of the prostate and surrounding tissue which need treatment and protect areas which do not need treatment; three-dimensional conformational therapy is a more sophisticated form of this method

Contracture
scarring which can occur at the bladder neck after a radical prostatectomy and which results in narrowing of the passage between the bladder and the urethra

Corpora Cavernosa
a part of a man's penis which fills with blood when he is sexually excited, giving the organ the stiffness required for intercourse

Corpora Spongiosum
a spongy chamber in a man's penis which fills with blood when he is sexually excited, giving the organ the stiffness required for intercourse

Cryoablation
(see Cryosurgery)

Cryosurgery
the use of liquid nitrogen probes to freeze a particular organ to extremely low temperatures to kill the tissue, including any cancerous tissue; when used to treat prostate cancer, the cryoprobes are guided by transrectal ultasound

Cryotherapy
(see Cryosurgery)

CT Scan, Computerized or Computed Tomography
(see Cat Scan)

Cyclophosphamide (Cytoxan)
an oral chemotherapy agent that can be used in the treatment of advanced prostate cancer

Cyproterone
an antiandrogen

Cystoscope
an instrument used by physicians to look inside the bladder and the urethra

Cystoscopy
the use of a cystoscope to look inside the bladder and the urethra

Cytokines
growth factors important to cellular function, they help normal and cancer cells grow

Debulking
reduction of the volume of cancer by one of several techniques; most frequently used to imply surgical debulking

DES
(see Diethylstilbestrol)

Dexamethasone (Decadron)
a high-dose steroid usually given if it is suspected that a patient may have a spinal cord compression

DHT
(see Dihydrotestosterone)

Diagnosis
the evaluation of signs, symptoms, and selected test results by a physician to determine the physical and biological causes of the signs and symptoms and whether a specific disease or disorder is involved

Diethylstilbestrol (DES)
a female hormone commonly used in treatment of prostate cancer

Differentiation
the use of the differences between prostate cancer cells when seen under the microscope as a method to grade the severity of the disease; well differentiated cells are easily recognized as normal cells, while poorly differentiated cells are abnormal, cancerous, and difficult to recognize as belonging to any particular type of cell group

Digital Rectal Examination
the use by a physician of a lubricated and gloved finger inserted into the rectum to feel for abnormalities of the prostate and rectum

Dihydrotestosterone
(DHT) (5 alpha-dihydrotestosterone) the male hormone which is most active in the prostate; it is manufactured when an enzyme (5 alpha reductase) in the prostate stimulates the transformation of testosterone to DHT

Diploid
having one complete set of normally paired chromosomes; i.e., a normal amount of DNA; diploid cancer cells tend to grow slowly and respond well to hormone therapy

DNA
Deoxyribonucleic Acid; the basic biologically active chemical which defines the physical development and growth of nearly all living organisms

Docetaxel (Taxotere)
A chemotherapy agent for hormone-refractory prostate cancer. It is a microtubule inhibitor. It is often used with estramustine

Double-Blind
a form of clinical trial in which neither the physician nor the patient know the actual treatment which any individual patient is receiving; double-blind trials are a way of minimizing the effects of the personal opinions of patients and physicians on the results of the trial

Doubling Time
the time that it takes a particular focus of cancer to double in size

Downsizing
the use of hormonal or other forms of management to reduce the volume of prostate cancer in and/or around the prostate prior to attempted curative treatment

Downstaging
the use of hormonal or other forms of management in the attempt to lower the clinical stage of prostate cancer prior to attempted curative treatment (e.g., from stage T3a to stage T2b); this technique is highly controversial

DRE
(see Digital Rectal Examination)

Dysplasia
(see PIN)

Dysuria
urination which is problematic or painful

Edema
swelling or accumulation of fluid in some part of the body

Ejaculatory Ducts
The tubular passages through which semen reaches the prostatic urethra during orgasm

Emcyt
the brand or trade name of estramustine phosphate in the United States

Endogenous
inherent, naturally to the organism

Erectile Dysfunction
(see Impotence)

Estramustine Phosphate
a chemotherapeutic agent used in the treatment of some patients with advanced prostate cancer

Estrogen
a female hormone; certain estrogens (e.g., diethylstilbestrol) are used by some physicians for treatment of prostate cancer

Etoposide
(VP-16, VePesid) an oral chemotherapy drug that is used for the treatment of hormone-refractory prostate cancer. It is used in conjunction with estramustine

Eulexin
the brand or trade name of flutamide in the United States

Experimental
an unproven (or even untested) technique or procedure; note that certain experimental treatments are commonly used in the mangement of prostate cancer

External Radiation Therapy (also External Beam Therapy)
a form of radiation therapy in which the radiation is delivered by a machine pointed at the area to be radiated

False Negative
an erroneous negative test result; for example, an imaging test that fails to show the presence of a cancer tumor, later found by biopsy, is said to have returned a false negative result

False Positive
a positive test result mistakenly identifying a state or condition that does not in fact exist

Finasteride
an inhibitor of the enzyme (5 alpha-reductase) that stimulates the conversion of testosterone to DHT; used to treat BPH

Flare Reaction
A temporary increase in tumor growth and symptoms caused by LHRH agonists; it can be mild to dangerous but may be prevented by taking an antiandrogen (generally Casodex or Eulexin) several days before starting LHRH agonist (Lupron or Zoladex)

Flow Cytometry
a measurement method that determines the fraction of cells that are diploid, tetraploid, aneuploid, etc.

Flutamide
(Eulexin) an antiandrogen used in the palliative hormonal treatment of advanced prostate cancer and

sometimes in the adjuvant and neoadjuvant hormonal treatment of earlier stages of prostate cancer; normal dosage is 2 capsules every 8 hours (not just at meals)

Frequency
the need to urinate often

Frozen Section
a technique in which removed tissue is frozen, cut into thin slices, and stained for microscopic examination; a pathologist can rapidly complete a frozen section analysis; for this reason it is commonly used during surgery to quickly provide the surgeon with vital information such as a preliminary pathologic opinion of the presence or absence of prostate cancer (usually in the pelvic lymph nodes)

Gastrointestinal
related to the digestive system and/or the intestines

Genital System
the biological system which (in males) includes the testicles, vas deferens, prostate, and penis

Genitourinary System
the combined genital and urinary systems; also known as the genitourinary tract

Gland
a structure or organ which produces a substance which is used in another part of the body

Gleason
name of physican who developed the Gleason grading system commonly used to grade prostate cancer

Gleason Score
a widely used method for classifying the cellular differentiation of cancerous tissues; the less the cancerous cells appear like normal cells, the more malignant the cancer; two numbers, each from 1-5, are assigned successively to the two most predominant patterns of differentiation present in the examined tissue sample and are added together to produce the Gleason score; high numbers indicate poor differentiation and therefore cancer

GNRH, Genadotropin-Releasing Hormone
(see LHRH Analogs)

Goserelin Acetate
a luteinizing hormone releasing hormone analog used in the palliative hormonal treatment of advanced prostate cancer and sometimes in the adjuvant and neoadjuvant hormonal treatment of earlier stages of prostate cancer

Grade
a means of describing the potential degree of severity of a cancer based on the appearance of cancer cells under a microscope (see Gleason Score)

Gynecomastia
enlargement or tenderness of the male breasts or nipples; a possible side effect of hormonal therapy

Hematospermia
the occurrence of blood in the semen

Hematuria
the occurence of blood in the urine

Hereditary
inherited from one's parents and earlier generations

Heredity
the historical distribution of biological characteristics through a group of related individuals via their DNA

Histology
the study of the appearance and behavior of tissue, usually carried out under a microscope by a pathologist (who is a physician) or a histologist (who is not necessarily a physician)

Hormone
biologically active chemicals that are responsible for many important body functions and the development of secondary sexual characteristics

Hormone Therapy
the use of hormones, hormone analogs, and certain surgical techniques to treat disease (in this case, advanced prostate cancer). The purpose of hormonal therapy in general is to lower testosterone to castrate or prepuberty levels. Hormones are used either on their own or in combination with other hormones or in combination with other methods of treatment; because prostate cancer is usually dependent on male hormones to grow, hormonal therapy can be an effective means of alleviating symptoms and retarding the development of the disease

Hot Flash
the sudden sensation of warmth in the face, neck, and upper body; a side effect of many forms of hormone therapy

Hypercalcemia
abnormally high concentrations of calcium in the blood, indicating leeching of calcium from bone (tumors raise serum calcium levels by destroying bone by releasing PTH or a PTH-like substance, osteoclast-activating factor, prostaglandins,and perhaps, a vitamin D-like sterol). Symptoms of hypercalcemia may include drowsiness, lethargy, headaches, depression or apathy, irritability, confusion, weakness, muscle flaccidity, bone pain, pathologic fractures, signs of heart block, cardiac arrest in systole, hypertension, anorexia, nausea, vomiting, constipation, dehydration, polydipsia, renal polyuria, flank pain, and eventually azotemia (excess of urea or other nitrogenous substances in the blood). Hypercalcemia is rare in prostate cancer

Hyperplasia
enlargement of an organ or tissue because of an increase in the number of cells in that organ or tissue; (see also Benign Prostatic Hypertrophy)

Hyperthermia
treatment that uses heat; for example, heat produced by microwave radiation

Imaging
a technique or method allowing a physician to see something which would not normally be visible. An x-ray, ultrasound, and ProstaScint scan are all examples of imaging techniques

Immune System
the biological system which protects a person or animal from the effects of foreign materials such as bacteria, cancer cells, and other things which might make that person or animal sick

Implant
a device that is inserted into the body; e.g., a tiny container of radioactive material inserted in or near a tumor; also a device inserted in order to replace

or substitute for an ability which has been lost; for example, a penile implant is a device which can be surgically inserted into the penis to provide rigidity for intercourse

Impotence
the inability to have or to maintain an erection

Incidental
insignificant or irrelevant; for example, incidental prostate cancer (also known as latent prostate cancer) is a form of prostate cancer which is of no clinical significance to the patient in whom it is discovered

Incontinence
(urinary incontinence) loss of urinary control; there are various kinds and degrees of incontinence; overflow incontinence is a condition in which the bladder retains urine after voiding; as a consequence, the bladder remains full most of the time, resulting in involuntary seepage of urine from the bladder; stress incontinence is the involuntary discharge of urine when there is increased pressure upon the bladder, as in coughing or straining to lift heavy objects; total incontinence is the inability to voluntarily exercise control over the sphincters of the bladder neck and urethra, resulting in total loss of retentive ability

Indication
a reason for doing something or taking some action; also used to mean the approved clinical application of a drug

Inflammation
any form of swelling or pain or irritation

Informed Consent
permission to proceed given by a patient after being fully informed of the purposes and potential consequences of a medical procedure

Interferon
a body protein that affects antibody production and can modulate (regulate) the immune system

Interstitial
within a particular organ; for example, interstitial prostate radiation therapy is radiation therapy

applied within the prostate using implanted radioactive pellets or seeds (see also Brachytherapy)

Intravenous
into a vein

Invasive
requiring an incision or the insertion of an instrument or substance into the body

Investigational
a drug or procedure allowed by the FDA for use in clinical trials

IVP, Intravenous Pyelogram
a procedure which introduces an x-ray absorbing dye into the urinary tract in order to allow the physician a superior image of the tract by taking an x-ray. This test is rarely used to check for the spread of cancer to the kidneys and bladder but is a common test done for other conditions besides prostate cancer

Kegel Exercises
a set of exercises designed to improve the strength of the muscles used in urinating

Ketoconazole (Nizoral)
a drug which can be used as a second-line hormonal agent when primary castration therapy fails

Kidney
one of a pair of organs whose primary function is to filter the fluids passing through the body

Laparoscopy
a technique which allows the physician to observe internal organs directly through a piece of optical equipment inserted directly into the body through a small surgical incision

Latent
insignificant or irrelevant; for example, latent prostate cancer (also known as incidental prostate cancer) is a form of prostate cancer which is of no clinical significance to the patient

Leuprolide Acetate
an LHRH analog

LHRH
(see Luteinizing Hormone Releasing Hormone)

LHRH Analogs (or Agonists)
synthetic compounds that are chemically similar to luteinizing hormone releasing hormone (LHRH), but are sufficiently different; they suppress testicular production of testosterone by binding to the LHRH receptor in the pituitary gland and either have no biological activity and therefore competitively inhibit the action of LHRH, or have LHRH activity that exhausts the production of LH by the pituitary; used in the palliative hormonal treatment of advanced prostate cancer and sometimes in the adjuvant and neoadjuvant hormonal treatment of earlier stages of prostate cancer

Libido
interest in sexual activity

LNCap
a line of human prostate cancer cells used in laboratory studies; this cell line is hormonally dependent

Lobe
one of the two sides of an organ which clearly has two sides (e.g., the prostate or the brain)

Localized
restricted to well-defined area

Lupron
the USA trade or brand name of Leuprolide Acetate, an LHRH agonist

Luteinizing Hormone Releasing Hormone (LHRH)
a hormone responsible for stimulating the production of testosterone in the body

Lymph (also Lymphatic Fluid)
the clear fluid in which all of the cells in the body are constantly bathed; carries cells that help fight infection

Lymph Nodes
the small glands which occur throughout the body and which filter the clear fluid known as lymph or lymphatic fluid; lymph nodes filter out bacteria and other toxins, as well as cancer cells

Lymphadenectomy
also known as a pelvic lymph node dissection, this procedure involves the removal and microscopic examination of selected lymph nodes, a common site of metastatic disease with prostate cancer; this procedure can be performed during surgery prior to the removal of the prostate gland, or by means of a small incision a "laparoscopic lymphadenectomy" may be performed, a simple operation requiring only an overnight stay in the hospital

Lymphatic System
the tissue and organs that produce, store, and carry cells that fight infection; includes bone marrow, spleen, thymus, lymph nodes, and channels that carry lymph fluid

MAB
Maximal Androgen Blockade (see CHT, CHB, ADT)

MAD
Maximal Androgen Deprivation (see ADT, CHB, CHT)

Magnetic Resonance
absorption of specific frequencies of radio and microwave radiation by atoms placed in a strong magnetic field.

Magnetic Resonance Imaging (MRI)
the use of magnetic resonance with atoms in body tissues to produce distinct cross-sectional, and even three-dimensional images of internal organs; MRI is primarily of use in staging biopsy-proven prostate cancer

Malignancy
a growth or tumor composed of cancerous cells

Malignant
cancerous; tending to become progressively worse and to result in death; having the invasive and metastatic (spreading) properties of cancer

Margin
normally used to mean the "surgical margin," which is the outer edge of the tissue removed during surgery; if the surgical margin shows no sign of cancer ("negative margins") the prognosis for cure is generally better than if the margins are positive.

Medical Oncologist
an oncologist primarily trained in the use of medicines (rather than surgery) to treat cancer

Megesterol Acetate
(Megace) a drug used to stimulate appetite in patients

Metastasize
spread of a malignant tumor to other parts of the body

Metastatic
having the characteristics of a secondary tumor

Metastatic Workup
a group of tests, including bone scans, x-rays, and blood tests, to determine whether cancer has metastasized

Metastron
the brand or trade name of Strontium-89 in the United States

Microtubules
scaffold-like structures in the cell that control cell division. Many chemotherapy drugs target the microtubules

Misstaging
the assignment of an incorrect clinical stage at initial diagnosis because of the difficulty of assessing the available information with accuracy

Mitosis
the process of a cell dividing into two cells. This is controlled by the microtubules (see Microtubules).

Mitoxantrone (Novantrone)
A chemotherapy drug for prostate cancer that has been shown to decrease pain when used in conjunction with prednisone (a steroid medicine). It is approved for this use in prostate cancer by the FDA.

Monoclonal
formed from a single group of identical cells; it can also refer to antibodies which only react to a single type of antigen

Morbidity
unhealthy consequences and complications resulting from treatment

MRI
(see Magnetic Resonance Imaging)

Negative
the term used to describe a test result which does not show the presence of the substance or material for which the test was carried out; for example, a negative bone scan would show no sign of bone metastases

Neoadjuvant
added before; for example, neoadjuvant hormone therapy is hormone therapy given prior to another form of treatment such as a radical prostatectomy

Neoplasia
the growth of cells under conditions that would tend to prevent the development of normal tissue (e.g., a cancer)

Nerve Sparing
term used to describe a type of prostatectomy in which the surgeon saves the nerves that effect sexual and related functions

Nilutamide
an antiandrogen

Nocturia
the need to urinate frequently at night

Noninvasive
not requiring any incision or the insertion of an instrument or substance into the body

NSE
neuron-specific enolase; a neuroendocrine marker (see CGA)

Oncologist
a physician who specializes in the treatment of various types of cancer

Oncology
the branch of medical science dealing with tumors; an oncologist is a specialist in the study of cancerous tumors

Orchiectomy
the surgical removal of the testicles

Organ
a group of tissues that work in concert to carry out a specific set of functions (e.g., the heart, lungs, or prostate)

Osteoblast
cell that forms bone

Osteoclast
cell that breaks down bone-cell, grows in bone tissue, and apparently absorbs bone tissue

Osteolysis
destruction of bone

Overstaging
the assignment of an overly high clinical stage at initial diagnosis because of the difficulty of assessing the available information with accuracy (e.g., stage T3b as opposed to stage T2b)

Paclitaxel (Taxol)
A commonly used chemotherapy agent for hormone-refractory prostate cancer. It is a microtubule inhibitor. It is often used with estramustine.

Palliative
designed to relieve a particular problem without necessarily solving it; for example, palliative therapy is given in order to relieve symptoms and improve quality of life, but does not cure the patient

Palpable
capable of being felt during a physical examination by an experienced physician; in the case of prostate cancer, this normally refers to some form of abnormality of the prostate which can be felt during a digital rectal examination

PAP (Prostatic Acid Phosphatase)
an enzyme now measured only rarely to decide whether prostate cancer has escaped from the prostate

Pathologist
a physician who specializes in the examination of tissues and blood samples to help decide which

diseases are present and how they should be treated

PDQ (Physicians Data Query)
a NCI supported database available to physicians, containing current information on standard treatments and ongoing clinical trials

Pelvis
that part of the skeleton that joins the lower limbs of the body together

Penile
of the penis

Penis
the male organ used in urination and intercourse

Perineal
of the perineum

Perineum
the area of the body between the scrotum and the rectum; a perineal procedure utilizes this area as the point of entry to the body

Perioheral
outside the central region

PET Scan
Positron emission tomography using a radioactive isotope that is taken up by tumor tissue showing that the tumor is functional; current studies do not indicate a high utility of PET scanning in prostate cancer that is newly diagnosed, perhaps related to the usual slow doubling times

PIN (Prostatic Intraepithelial [or Intraductal] Neoplasia)
a pathologically identifiable condition believed to be a possible precursor of prostate cancer, also known more simply as dysplasia by many physicans

Placebo
a form of safe but nonactive treatment frequently used as a basis for comparison with drugs in research studies

Ploidy
a term used to describe the number of sets of chromosomes in a cell (see also Diploid and Aneuploid)

Positive
the term used to describe a test result which shows the presence of the substance or material for which the test was carried out; for example, a positive bone scan would show signs of bone metastases

Posterior
the rear; for example, the posterior of the prostate faces a man's back

Prednisone
a steroid medicine that is often used in advanced prostate cancer as a single agent or in combination with other medicines

Prognosis
the patient's potential clinical outlook based on the status and probable course of his disease; chance of recovery

Progression
continuing growth or regrowth of the cancer

Prolactin
(PRL) a trophic hormone produced by the pituitary that increases androgen receptors, increases sensitivity to androgens, and regulates production and secretion of citrate

Proscar
brand name of finasteride

ProstaScint
a monoclonal antibody test directed against the Prostate Specific Membrane Antigen (PSMA); seems to focus on androgen-independent tumor tissue

Prostate
the gland surrounding the urethra and immediately below the bladder in males

Prostatectomy
surgical removal of part or all of the prostate gland

Prostate-Specific Antigen
(see PSA)

Prostate - Specific Membrane Antigen (PSMA)
PSMA is a protein that is found on the membranes of prostate cells. This antibody forms the basis of the ProstaScint test (see Monoclonal)

Prostatic Acid Phosphatase
(see PAP)

Prostatitis
infection or inflammation of the prostate gland treatable by medication and/or manipulation; (BPH is a more permanent laying down of fibroblasts and connective tissue caused when the prostate tries to contain a relatively silent chronic lower-grade infection, often requiring a TURP to relieve the symptoms)

Prosthesis
a man-made device used to replace a normal body part or function

Protocol
a precise set of methods by which a research study is to be carried out

PSA (Prostate-Specific Antigen)
a protein secreted by the epithelial cells of the prostate gland including cancer cells; an elevated level in the blood indicates an abnormal condition of the prostate gland, either benign or malignant; it is used to detect potential problems in the prostate gland and to follow the progress of PCa Therapy (see Screening)

PSA-II
(Prostate-Specific Antigen Type II Assay), reports the percentage of free-PSA to total-PSA (total PSA = free PSA + bound PSA); helpful for screening purposes when PSA values are above the normal threshold for an age group and less than 10; one study showed that men with PSA II > 25% had no PCa; those with <10 % were likely to have PCa; not yet FDA approved (4/96), but available

PSA RT-PCR
(PSA, Reverse Transcriptase, Polymerase Chain Reaction), a blood test that detects micrometastatic cells circulating in the bloodstream; may be useful as a screening tool to help avoid unnecessary invasive treatments (RP, RT etc.) for patients with metastasized PCa; not FDA approved (4/96),but available at locations where FDA approved clinical trials of the test are being conducted

Quality of Life
an evaluation of health status relative to the patient's age, expectations, and physical and mental capabilities

Radiation Oncologist
a physician who has received special training regarding the treatment of cancers with different types of radiation

Radiation Therapy (RT)
the use of x-rays and other forms of radiation to destroy malignant cells and tissue

Radical
(in a surgical sense) directed at the cause of a disease; thus radical prostatectomy is the surgical removal of the prostate with the intent to cure the problem believed to be caused by or within the prostate

Radical Prostatectomy
an operation to remove the entire prostate gland and seminal vesicles

Radioisotope
a type of atom (or a chemical which is made with a type of atom) that emits radioactivity

Radio Sensitivity
the degree to which a type of cancer responds to radiation therapy

Radiotherapy
(see Radiation Therapy)

Randomized
the process of assiging patients to different forms of treatment in a research study in a random manner

Rectal Exam
(see Digital Rectal Exam)

Rectum
the final part of the intestines which ends at the anus

Recurrence
the reappearance of disease

Refractory
resistant to therapy; e.g., hormone-refractory

prostate cancer is resistant to forms of treatment based on the use of hormones

Regression
reduction in the size of a single tumor or reduction in the number and/or size of several tumors

Remission
the real or apparent disappearance of some or all of the signs or symptoms of cancer; the period (temporary or permanent) during which a disease remains under control, without progressing; even complete remission does not necessarily indicate cure

Resection
surgical removal

Resectoscope
instrument inserted through the urethra used by a urologist to remove tissue (usually from the prostate) while the physician can actually see precisely where he is cutting

Resistance
(in a medical sense) a patient's ability to fight off a disease as a result of the effectiveness of the patient's immune system

Response
a decrease in disease that occurs because of treatment

Retention
difficulty in initiation of urination or the inability to completely empty the bladder

Retropubic Prostatectomy
surgical removal of the prostate through an incision in the abdomen

Risk
the chance or probability that a particular event will or will not happen

RP
(see Radical Prostatectomy)

RTCPR
(see RT-PCR)

RT-PCR
(Reverse Transcriptase, Polymerase Chain Reaction), a technique which allows a physician to search for tiny quantities of protein, such as PSA, in the blood or other fluids and tissues; (see PSA, RT-PCR)

Salvage
a procedure intended to "rescue" a patient following the failure of a prior treatment; for example, a salvage prostatectomy would be the surgical removal of the prostate after the failure of prior radiation therapy or cryosurgery

Screening
to separate patients with tumors from those without tumors; multiple criteria are often used; the following PSA screening "cutoff" levels for PCa are replacing the older 4.0 value:
Age PSA "cutoff"
40-49 up to 2.5
50-59 up to 3.5
60-69 up to 4.5
70-79 up to 6.5

Scrotum
the pouch of skin containing a man's testicles

Secondary To
derived from or consequent to a primary event or thing

Selenium
a relatively rare nonmetallic element found in food in small quantities which may have some effect in prevention of cancer

Semen
the whitish, opaque fluid emitted by a male at ejaculation

Seminal
related to the semen; for example, the seminal vesicles are glands at the base of the bladder and connected to the prostate that provide nutrients for the semen

Sensitivity
the probability that a diagnostic test can correctly identify the presence of a particular disease assuming the proper conduct of the test;specifically, the number of true positive results divided by the sum of the true positive results and the false negative results (see Specificity)

Sextant
having six parts; thus, a sextant biopsy is a biopsy that takes six samples

Side Effect
a reaction to a medication or treatment (most commonly used to mean an unnecessary or undesirable effect)

Sign
physical changes that can be observed as a consequence of an illness or disease

Specificity
the probability that a diagnostic test can correctly identify the absence of a particular disease assuming the proper conduct of the test; specifically, the number of true negative results divided by the sum of the true negative results and the false positive results; a method that detects 95% of true PCa cases is highly sensitive, but if it also falsely indicates that 40% of those who do not have PCa do have PCa, then its specificity is 60%; rather poor

Spinal cord
the group of nerves that runs down the middle of your back. These are protected by your back bones (vertebral bodies)

Spinal Cord Compression
this occurs when prostate cancer spreads to the spine and it invades the spinal cord. This usually results in pain or tingling shooting down the legs. This is a medical emergency and you should go to an emergency room immediately.

Spine
all of the backbones

Stage
a term used to define the size and physical extent of a cancer

Staging
the process of assigning a stage in a specific patient in light of all the available information; it is used to help determine appropriate therapy; there

are two staging methods: the Whitmore–Jewett staging classification (1956) and the more detailed TNM (Tumor, Nodes, Metastases) classification (1998) of the American Joint Committee on Cancer and the International Union Against Cancer. Staging should be subcategorized as clinical staging and pathologic staging. Pathologic stage usually relates to what is found at the time of surgery.

Stent
a tube used by a surgeon to drain fluids

Stricture
scarring as a result of a procedure or an injury that constricts the flow of urine through the urethra

Strontium-89 (Metaszron)
an injectable radioactive product that is used to relieve bone pain for some patients with prostate cancer which no longer responds to hormones or appropriate forms of chemotherapy

Subcapsular
under the capsule; for example, a subcapsular orchiectomy is a form of castration in which the contents of each testicle is removed but the testicular capsules are then closed and remain in the scrotum

Suramin
an experimental drug

Suture
surgical stitching used in the closure of a cut or incision

Symptom
a feeling, sensation, or experience associated with or resulting from a physical or mental disorder and noticeable by the patient

Systemic
throughout the whole body

Testicle
(see Testis)

Testis
one of two male reproductive glands located inside the scrotum which are the primary sources of the male hormone testosterone

Testosterone (T)
the male hormone or androgen which comprises most of the androgens in a man's body; chiefly produced by the testicles; may be produced in tissues from precursors such as androstenedione; T is essential to complete male sexual function and fertility

Therapy
the treatment of disease or disability

TNM
(Tumor, Nodes, Metastases) (see Staging)

Transition
change; for example, the transition zone of the prostate is the area of the prostate closest to the urethra and has features which distinguish it from the much larger peripheral zone

Transperineal
through the perineum

Transrectal
through the rectum

Transurethral
through the urethra

Treatment
administration of remedies to patient for a disease

TRUS
Transrectal Ultrasound; a method that uses echoes of ultrasound waves (far beyond the hearing range) to image the prostate by inserting an ultasound probe into the rectum; commonly used to visualize prostate biopsy procedures

TRUS-P
(see TRUS)

Tumor
an excessive growth of cells caused by uncontrolled and disorderly cell replacement; an abnormal tissue growth that can be either benign or malignant (see Benign, Malignant)

TURP (Transurethral Resection of the Prostate)
a surgical procedure to remove tissue obstructing the urethra; the technique involves the insertion of

an instrument called a resectoscope into the penile urethra, and is intended to relieve obstruction of urine flow due to enlargement of the prostate

TUR/P
(see TURP)

Ultrasound
sound waves at a particular frequency (far beyond the hearing range) whose echoes bouncing off tissue can be used to image internal organs (e.g., a baby in the womb)

Understaging
the assignment of an overly low clinical stage at initial diagnosis because of the difficulty of assessing the available information with accuracy (e.g., stage T2b as opposed to stage T3b)

Unit
a surgical term for a pint (usually of blood)

Ureter
an anatomical tube that drains urine from one of the two kidneys to the bladder

Urethra
the tube that drains urine from the bladder through the prostate and out through the penis

Urgency
the need to urinate very soon

Urinary System
the group of organs and their interconnections that permits excess, filtered fluids to exit the body, including (in the male) the kidneys, the ureters, bladder, urethra, and penis

Urologist
a doctor trained first as a surgeon who specializes in disorders of the genitourinary system

UTI
urinary tract infection; an infection identifiable by the presence of bacteria (or theoretically, viruses) in the urine; may be associated with a fever or a burning sensation on urination

Vas Deferens
tube through which sperm travels from the testes to the prostate prior to ejaculation

Vasectomy
operation to make a man sterile by cutting the vas deferens, thus preventing passage of sperm from the testes to the prostate

Vertebral bodies
your individual backbones. They hold you erect and protect your spinal cord

Vesicle
a small sac containing a biologically important fluid

Vinblastine (Velban)
A chemotherapy agent that attacks the microtubules. Often used with estramustine

Watchful Waiting
active observation and regular monitoring of a patient without actual treatment

Whitmore-Jewett Staging
(see Staging)

X-Ray
a type of high energy radiation that can be used at low levels to make images of the internal structures of the body and at high levels for radiation therapy

Zoladex
trade or brand name for goserelin acetate, a LHRH agonist

Zone
part or area of an organ